HIV on TV

HIV on TV

Popular Culture's Epidemic

Malynnda A. Johnson

LEXINGTON BOOKS
Lanham • Boulder • New York • London

Published by Lexington Books
An imprint of The Rowman & Littlefield Publishing Group, Inc.
4501 Forbes Boulevard, Suite 200, Lanham, Maryland 20706
www.rowman.com

Unit A, Whitacre Mews, 26-34 Stannary Street, London SE11 4AB

British Library Cataloguing in Publication Information Available

Library of Congress Cataloging-in-Publication Data Available

ISBN 978-1-4985-4726-0 (cloth : alk. paper)
ISBN 978-1-4985-4727-7 (electronic)

∞™ The paper used in this publication meets the minimum requirements of American National Standard for Information Sciences Permanence of Paper for Printed Library Materials, ANSI/NISO Z39.48-1992.

Printed in the United States of America

This book is wholeheartedly dedicated to my loving friends who are living each day with a virus many still do not care to understand. You have inspired me beyond words.

Contents

Introduction

In 1987 it was "killing all the right people" (*Designing Women*), by the nineties it might not kill you but your professional career would soon be over; today "HIV is the new diabetes, it's just another chronic illness" (*Nip/Tuck*). Across decades HIV narratives have shaped the perceptions and understanding viewers have about the virus. In a time where talking about sex is still taboo from an educational standpoint, but not from a commercial one, television's continued use of HIV as a dramatic or comedic storyline offers two distinct possibilities. First is the opportunity to educate and correct misperceptions. Countless shows have successfully embedded health messages about HIV in their storylines raising awareness and providing facts. One such example, is *Grey's Anatomy*'s inclusion of the reality that with proper precautions there is a 90 percent chance an HIV-infected mother can give birth to an HIV-negative baby. While working closely with medical organizations can improve the quality of the message, far fewer shows have chosen to do to so. For some shows the messages, characters, and situations used to bring up the topic of HIV have contributed to raising awareness about a virus few want to talk about. However, it is apparent that when HIV is used as a devise simply to create conflict, or a laugh, dangerous misperceptions and miseducation occur. By only showing certain populations contracting the virus, a consistent lack of consequences when risky behaviors take place, as well as falling back on stereotypes and discrimination as the foundation for a punchline, viewers are continuously fed information perpetuating fear, stigma, and the belief that safer sex practices are not really needed. Thus, impinging on the prevention efforts of a now completely preventable virus.

While there remains to be a cure for the human immunodeficiency virus (HIV) a great wealth of knowledge has been collected. We now understand how it is passed from person to person, and we understand that while it is often found in certain demographics everyone engaging in risky behaviors is in danger. Testing is often free and takes less than an hour in most clinics, and tools for prevention are easy to find. Yet regardless of the knowledge people have about the virus, the perception remains, it will never happen to me. The question is, why?

Generally speaking, people tend to believe that they are immune or invulnerable to events or consequences.[1] When it comes to the consequences of unprotected sex, a large majority of people seem to only focus on the issue of unplanned pregnancy. As discussed later in the book young people specifically do not identify HIV as a risk they need to be concerned with. Not only are young people not concerned about their risk, many stereotypes and stigmas about those living with the virus remain in play. Again, the question is, why? This book argues that in part this is due to the manner though which HIV has been portrayed in the media.

Given the ongoing dismantling and outright obstruction of comprehensive sex education classes in the United States, for many television serves as one of the only means of providing facts about the virus. For some writers, including a narrative about HIV within a show is a direct attempt to pick up the burden of educating audiences, left by an absent government. Other writers, simply observed the instant attention the virus creates whenever it was mentioned in the media. The problem, however, is audiences rarely question the messages being presented unless the topic is one in which they already personally identify with. Without taking a critical eye to the messages presented it is easy to believe that HIV only impacts certain groups. A storyline created and continued since the very beginning.

A BRIEF HISTORY OF HIV

The year was 1981, and news outlets were calling it the gay plague, gay cancer, and eventually even gay-related immune deficiency (GRID). Upon discovering that the virus killing thousands was not limited to gay populations, HIV and acquired immunodeficiency syndrome (AIDS) became the official terms. Yet regardless of the official titles, given the manner through which media outlets had framed HIV and AIDS the fear, stigma, and unease HIV and AIDS generated in the 80s has in many ways continued, 35 years later.

Over the last three and a half decades countless celebrities have spoken out and passed away from the virus. Charity galas, concerts, movies, and television shows have each taken their turn raising awareness and funds for research. Presidents and politicians have come together and fought over the role government should play in the prevention of an illness often thought to be brought on by one's own actions. Thankfully, with medical advancements and research what is understood about HIV and AIDS far surpasses the questions still unanswered. Unfortunately, the advancements of rapid testing and medical treatments have only encouraged people to become complacent, forgetting the pandemic still plaguing an estimated 1.2 million people in the United States (CDC 2014) and 36.7 million worldwide.

Although the number of young adults reporting to be sexually active appears to have declined, the Centers for Disease Control (CDC) report that 44,073 new cases of HIV were reported in the United States last year, young adults, especially adolescent males, accounting for three-quarters of new diagnoses (CDC 2014). Young adults' risk for HIV is also compounded given the large number (approximately one in four) testing positive for sexually transmitted diseases each year (CDC 2014). Considering the time span between contracting HIV and exhibiting clinical symptoms, coupled with the fact that many young adults engage in behavior that places them at risk, such as inconsistent condom use, drinking alcohol and other drug use, the number of infected young adults may be underestimated (Lewis, Miguez-Burbano & Malow 2009; Ashenhurst, Wilhite, Harden, & Fromme 2017).

Despite the statistics surrounding HIV, and other sexually transmitted infections (STIs), the majority of young adults report not being concerned about the potential of becoming infected (Johnson 2015; Polacek et al. 2007; Vermund & Wilson 2002). One explanation for this phenomenon is that knowledge about HIV and AIDS is not translated into accurate estimates of risk (Albert & Steinberg 2011; Ellen et al. 2002; Foster et al. 2012). Be it the lack of interpersonal communication, stigma surrounding HIV, or a disparity of knowledge, young adults appear to have become complacent, not only in their behaviors, but also in their perceptions of risk. Thanks to political, religious, and educational red tape many young people are not acquiring accurate education about sexual health. Therefore, the question is, where do young people acquire their perceptions of risk for HIV? Short of someone encountering a family member or friend living with HIV, media may convey the only messages about risk; thus forming the foundations of understanding severity and susceptibility.

CONSTRUCTING HIV AND AIDS

Over the years, HIV has been presented and discussed through a variety of metaphors, news headlines, characters, and narratives. Each mention of HIV in the media adds layer upon layer of understanding, ultimately constructing what is known about the virus. As explained by the theory of social representation, individuals gather most of their information about unknown phenomena from the mass media, which results in the first steps of forming public opinion (Morgan, Harrison, Chewning, Davis, & DiCorcia 2007). Given the nearly 8.5 hours young adults spend engaged with media it is important for research to examine the effect television media can have on viewers. While many forms of media, including print, radio, or the internet, contain messages focusing on sex and HIV, research suggests that the messages mediated through prime-time television are relatively more consistent than these other mediums (Brown, L'Engle, Pardun, Guo, Kenneavy, & Jackson 2006).

In his book *The AIDS Movie,* Kylo-Patrick Hart (2014) argues that the movies about AIDS were not *reflections* of society but more so *constructions*. Lessons presented on television construct, or shape, our perceptions of illness and form our understanding of the issue. Conrad and Barker (2010) argue that our attitudes toward, and knowledge of, health issues are embedded with cultural meaning that is not directly derived from the nature of the condition. As a result, cultural constructions shape how society responds to the illness itself as well as those living with it.

While narratives involving HIV are not as common as other health-related storylines, when young adults are asked where their HIV knowledge has come from they often state that most of what they know is gained through television (Beck, Pollard, & Greenberg, 2000; Johnson 2013). As such, Entertainment-Education (E-E) can be seen as an important strategy for incorporating health and other educational messages into popular entertainment media. When E-E is utilized it draws on viewers' emotional investment in television shows in the attempt to positively change awareness, knowledge, attitudes, and/or behaviors on specific issues (Kaiser Family Foundation 2006). Incorporating an educational message into popular entertainment content has the potential to raise awareness, increase knowledge, create favorable attitudes, and ultimately motivate people to take socially responsible action in their own lives (Singhal & Rogers 2002; Singhal & Rogers 2012). On the other hand, when behaviors or health conversations are included without educational strategy in mind, miseducation can occur.

Many of the current storylines use sex in terms of building dramatic effect and increasing ratings, rather than ensuring viewers are gaining valuable knowledge such as talking to doctors about HIV and STIs or negotiating the use of condoms with their partners. Additionally, the majority of popular television shows have neglected to include characters talking to a peer or partner about testing for STIs or HIV, nor have these shows provided a framework to highlight how conversations about safe sex might occur. By not attending to how HIV or safe sex is being framed, many of these shows may actually be contributing to, if not creating, misperceptions about the risk of HIV.

From HIV-positive characters to the emotions evoked throughout the storylines, HIV in popular culture provides a series of cultural constructions. When used to disseminate facts about HIV and AIDS, television media is able to educate audiences, reaching vast combinations of demographic backgrounds. Yet far too often, shows are less interested in the educational aspects, and more focused on the ratings received by including a controversial topic. Given the manner through which HIV is acquired it is considered taboo and a difficult conversation for many to engage in. However, media's framing of the virus has in many ways presented HIV as a semantic epidemic. As a result, it is possible that the way HIV has been discussed in headlines and narrative plots has perpetuated stigma, miseducated audiences, and encouraged the perception that only "some" are at risk.

Through the critical examination of over a hundred television shows, made-for-television movies, and interviews with actors portraying HIV-positive characters *HIV on TV: Popular Culture's Epidemic* presents how HIV has been discussed throughout the life of the virus. While HIV has remained a popular topic of research in many areas, such as stigma, social support, and barriers to testing, studies examining the cultural construction of one's perceptions of HIV through popular media have remained few in number. In fact, to date only a small handful of texts have examined HIV or AIDS in the media, and all were published in the mid- to late 90s. Therefore, I hope this book will improve the current understanding of how media has framed HIV, and help refocus the frames used when discussing sexual health topics. Additionally, I seek to create a potential template for understanding how other illnesses may be socially constructed through television media. HIV and AIDs are not the only health topics media writers weave in without education in mind. Countless shows have explored lifelong illnesses, such as mental illness, as a means of creating drama. The model used for this book provides a means through which other examinations could occur. Finally, by utilizing both rhetorical and qualitative methods, this book bridges a methodical gap and offers a new approach to applied research. Overall, my primary concern is understanding the role news, drama, and even comedic constructions have had in the continued advancement of HIV.

In order to unpack the education provided on the topic of HIV, and to understand how the virus has been constructed by the media, this book has been broken down into four sections. Part one provides the theoretical structures that underpin the analysis used throughout the book. In order to discern how media can serve as an educational tool, it is vital to first learn the theoretical frameworks explaining how mediated narratives function. Thus, the first chapter seeks to illuminate the *how* and *why* entertainment can function as an educational tool. As with learning about any historical or social event, multiple perspectives and frames must be taken into consideration. Therefore, chapter two shifts gears from the focus of teacher to one of critic. This chapter discusses the multiple meanings and rhetorical situations surrounding HIV while offering an argument for the importance of considering the genre used to frame the topic.

Part Two then presents the analysis of 35 years of HIV narratives found in news stories, and the dramatic and comedic shows. Chapter three offers the context surrounding the shows later examined. By highlighting news headlines during the three and a half decades of HIV (1980s, 90s, and 2000–now) themes surrounding the tone and viewpoint are identified. These frames provide an important background required to understand the ways in which the shows were responding to cultural events. Delving into the narratives themselves, the two genres of television, dramatic and comedic, are examined beginning with the first ever mentions of HIV and progressing to the modern examples of today. Each chapter examines critical choices and narrative constructions presented within the episodes.

Moving from the larger themes identified within the shows to the individual characters, part three explores the HIV/AIDS Body and impact of the portrayals of HIV on television. This section first offers an analysis of the HIV/AIDS-positive characters on television, and then shifts to the perspectives of the actors who have played them. Here the goal is to look deeper into some of the specific lessons presented in the shows by looking across both genres and time. Understanding that lessons presented on television are limited to what the viewers identify, the final chapter of part three offers the incite and voices from two groups of viewers. Finally, pulling together the lessons within the shows and perceptions of viewers, the final chapter offers suggestions for the future of HIV on television.

NOTE

1. Perloff, Linda S. "Social comparison and illusions of invulnerability to negative life events." In *Coping with negative life events*, pp. 217–242. Boston: Springer, 1987.

1

Teaching HIV

Chapter One

Television as Teacher

Lessons about HIV/AIDS have come in many forms over the years. As discussed in the introduction, narratives within certain genres share a common pedagogic function, such as news reports and educational movies. In such genres, the narratives are researched and strategically crafted seeking to educate the viewer, informing them of the risks and realities of the topic at hand. However, while these direct forms of education are helpful in raising awareness, they are not the only means. In fact, any time a character or message about HIV is embedded in a program the ability to shape perceptions of the viewer is possible.

For generations entertainment has been found to have a powerful ability to teach viewers. Beginning with narratives told with the goal of teaching, the chapter explores entertaining educational and didactic rhetoric. Highlighting two examples of how made-for-television movies and after school specials have overtly sought to educate viewers about HIV/AIDS. Yet it must be noted that HIV/AIDS education has never been restricted to pedagogically created narratives. Shows are thought to transport viewers into their screens. Characters whom audiences connect with provide a means for shaping the ideas and perceptions of viewers. Therefore, this chapter explores how modern lessons about HIV are often masked within the shows viewers are currently invested in; providing a platform for dissemination without suspicion from the audience. Ultimately, even though the intention of a show might not be to teach the viewer, it's crucial to understand that anytime HIV/AIDS enters a narrative, social and cultural lessons can be learned.

TELEVISION AS EDUCATOR

Media research has suggested that television viewers learn more from the media when they do not know much about the topic at hand (Dutta-Bergman 2004). In particular, a person's level of involvement with certain issues has been found to be a significant determinant of shaping their perception after being exposed to television content (Borchers 2012). As a result, even without consciously thinking about the information presented, passive learning is possible.

The use of narratives to teach audiences began far before the invention of the television (Hinyard & Kreuter 2007). Glik, Nowak, Valenete, Sapsis, & Martin (2002) argued that consistently well-designed and executed live theater performances are able to engage audiences, influencing the knowledge, attitudes, and behaviors of audience members. Additionally, they found that these shows positively impacted peer, social, and cultural norms. Developing this further, Gilk, Nowak, Valenete, Sapsis, & Martin, note that dramatic performances are linked to short-term gains in knowledge and noted for positive attitudes about health issues among audience members.

Used to encourage behavioral and social change Entertainment Education (E-E) is an important communication strategy with a goal to increase awareness and knowledge of a variety of topics (Asbeek, Fransen & Smit 2015). E-E aims to positively influence attitudes and/or behaviors through the shows in which viewers are already invested (Singhal & Rogers 2002). Historically, some of the first examples of E-E; the ability to teach lessons through means of entertainment, were the lessons taught within the stories of the Brothers Grimm (Tatar 1992). Brothers Grimm themselves argued, "fairy-tales offer good teaching, an application to the present, and they yield themselves so easily, thus provoking such moral lessons" (McGlathery 1993, 37). Through the use of sarcasm and violence, cleverly camouflaged within childlike tropes, their stories offered not only entertainment but also cultural and moral lessons.

In many ways fables and fairy-tale stories have influenced generations of children, teaching tales of not only princesses and pumpkins but also of hierarchies and cultural norms of their time. The frames these stories enacted offered an intriguing infrastructure for any educator seeking to shape young minds. Take for example the original tale of Goldilocks. Seeking to teach readers the importance of self-control, the dangers of entering homes without permission, and the harm that can be incurred from individual actions, the original version of the popular tale ends with papa bear eating the golden-haired child.

Seeing the potential of educating audiences through narratives, educators and filmmakers partnered together in the late 1940s to create a number of educational and entertaining films to be shown in the classroom. Conceived as being preventive medicine for young behaviors, tragic tales were told as means of terrifying viewers into conformity. Thus the "Mental Hygiene" films were created to shape the behavior of viewers by showing the impact certain behaviors or choices can have on one's life. In essence, "the videos visually spanked viewers with an assortment of cinematic paddles" (Smith 1999). While the creators of these films were drawn to the power entertainment had on students, they alleged a shared desire to guide young people toward behaviors that they felt would make them happier and more civically connected.

Discussing topics such as dating, physical hygiene, sex, drugs, and alcohol use, each video focused tightly on the message at hand showing a perfect world when rules were followed. To achieve such a perfect world, each storyline highlighted the praise of conformity, and the consequences of rebellion. The mental hygiene videos become wildly popular as teaching tools, not because they showed the world as it actually was, but because they showed life the way those in power wanted it to be (Smith 1999). As a result, responsibility was never shown as equal. Teens, and young adults were always at fault, and parents always played the savior or punisher role.

What made the mental hygiene videos successful, originally, was the clear messaging. However, researchers have since gleaned that the message alone was not enough (Singhal, Cody, Rodgers & Sabido 2003). Lessons presented within a movie or show should be direct and simple, however, they also need to be relatable and clearly show how the desired behavior would look in action. For nearly two decades mental hygiene videos served as powerful educational tools (Besley 2002). However, as the new generation's perceptions evolved more contemporary approaches were needed. Messages now need to be less obvious, and the context of the situations and behaviors needed to include more complexity. The ability to more acutely camouflage the moral lesson requires the use of didactic rhetoric.

DIDACTIC GENRES AND ENTERTAINMENT EDUCATION

The careful use of a speech, drama, or narrative with the goal of teaching a larger lesson can be classified as didactic rhetoric. Didactic rhetoric is a common genre in American discourse, shaping audience's expectations and understanding of a wide variety of topics. One of the most common forms of didactic rhetoric found today are the many social and cultural narratives found in television.

What Makes a Show Didactic?

Didactic, and E-E, genres specifically seek to both entertain and educate, and while many shows including a theme of health may appear to fit within this genre, before this distinction can be made, specific criteria must be applied. First is the examination of the use of theme. Smiley (1971) postulates there must be a distinction between didactic and mimetic, or performance-driven dramas, with the variation found in the way that the theme is employed. To be considered didactic, this theme should operate in two ways: it must be the dominant material for the character, but, more importantly, it must be the organizing thesis. In other words, the intended message must not only be at the forefront, but all other sub-messages should lead back to the primary theme. The second condition is that the narrative must evoke emotion. Without an emotional response, the lessons are more likely to be left behind once the narrative is complete. When audience members are able to become emotionally connected with a story, play, or show, then the audience members are more likely to become transported into the show, and will likely take away the new frame of reference (Moyer-Guse 2008).

The third and final condition for didactic rhetoric is the power of providing truth. This ability to provide truth is why medical accuracy of a show must be closely examined; thereby identifying the accuracy of information about HIV being portrayed. Research has already identified that young adults, and adults alike, learn most of what they know from the media (Dutta-Bergman 2004; Ruppel 2016), and therefore special attention must be paid to the information presented and what inferences the audience might make.

Albeit many of narratives examined for this book would likely not be classified as didactic, given the intention to educate was not always the primary goal, in 1992 Paramount Studios created a celebrity-filled "after school special" targeted at young adults. *Time Out: The Truth about HIV, AIDS, and You* merged a clear educational message that celebrities' young views would know. Overall the special provides an excellent example of a didactic narrative with the theme of raising viewers understanding of HIV.

The central lesson presented in the special is that HIV can happen to anyone, but most importantly is preventable. From the lips of one of the most famous people living with HIV, Magic Johnson tells viewers that he too thought the virus could never happen to him. Echoing the message singer Paula Abdul, teen actor Neil Patrick Harris, and many more speak directly to the viewer with facts and statistics from the Centers for Disease Control and the World Health Organization. While the overall feeling to the video is upbeat, with the use of bright colors and music, the tone throughout remains serious. Including the personal narratives of six young adults living with HIV.

The use of both celebrities as well as everyday people enhances the emotional connection for the audience. As discussed later in this chapter, the ability for a viewer to personally connect with a speaker greatly impacts the likelihood of a message sticking with the viewer. What *Time Out* does well is the inclusion of non-celebrities with various social and racial backgrounds.

Each speaker furthers the ideas presented by the celebrities within their tales of contracting HIV. Following the same emotionally, and largely fear-driven, formatting of the mental hygiene videos, Kimberly shares her journey with HIV. Kimberly states her life was pretty normal until she was fourteen, when she started becoming popular. She continues explaining that with new friends she soon started lying to her parents and doing things she knew her parents wouldn't support including engaging in unprotected sex. Years later, Kimberly discovered that not only was she HIV positive, but she had also passed the virus to her daughter.

Although *Time Out* provides a wealth of important facts about HIV, three significant limitations need to be addressed. First, is that none of the speakers are high school or even college age. Considering the music, graphics, and choices in celebrities the target audience is clearly young adults; however, they rarely see themselves on the screen. In only about 10 minutes of the hour-long special is a group of college age students shown. The behaviors discussed are framed as occurring during those times, but it is possible that younger viewers would still feel unable to personally identify with these stories.

A second limitation found was the use of fear appeals within the non-celebrity monologues. "The doctor told me I have HIV, and it is lethal," "The doctors tell me if I don't take care of myself, and take my meds, that I have a year or so to live. But that's just the doctors. Jesus is telling me something different," "I have watched a lot of my friends stop talking to me." Coming from these speakers these types of comments highlight the personal fears viewers have. To use fear campaigns effectively there needs to be a balance of information, fear, and action. The fear message cannot be left unsupported by means for the viewer to prevent that event from occurring. Within the *Time Out* special, some efficacy is presented, but not always in the right places.

Finally, this special is direct and in the viewer's face about the messages they present. There is no question about what the creators want viewers to think. Although the special offered a counternarrative to the typical, abstinence-only focus on "just don't have sex," the message being so concentrated is likely to come across as preachy and too educational. In other words though using a central persuasive route ensures the message is clear for the viewer such messages are easy to brush off.

Overall, *Time Out* can be argued as meeting each of the three requirements for didactic rhetoric. The central theme of raising knowledge and awareness of HIV is presented from multiple angles. Emotional appeals occur within the tone and personal testimonies, and countless myths of HIV are dispelled with the inclusion of facts and statistics. However, as discovered with viewers ignoring the messages within mental hygiene videos of the past, the direct health messages in after school specials are easily ignored. Understanding this challenge, health promoters in the mid- to late 90s began working directly with television writers and producers. Partnering with television writers has essentially served as a means of hiding the vegetables, in this case health messages, within the shows viewers already love.

TEACHING THROUGH TRANSPORTATION

O'Donnell (2016) argues that viewers do more than simply watch a program—they absorb it. By doing so, audiences become more than just viewers; they become involved with the medium, caring about what happens and even interacting with the characters by talking to the show. As a result, organizations around the world have partnered with television media outlets to create and insert storylines raising awareness of various health issues (Singhal & Rogers 2012).

Designing programs with health messages embedded in a show combines the power of mass media with a social model allowing observers to learn without the hazards and pain of personally experiencing an illness or situation (McKee, Bertrand, Becker-Benton, & Becker 2004). Moreover, by integrating messages about HIV and AIDS into the programs that viewers already watch, and more importantly are talking about, there is a greater chance of the messages impacting attitude and behavior. Not only does E-E offer an opportunity to increase awareness, but when the audience of an E-E program connects with a show, they often gain new opinions of the issue presented. Learning through observing, be it mediated or based on personal observation, occurs regardless of the intention behind the message. Meaning that regardless of the writer's goal to educate an audience about a health topic by including the topic in the first place, a viewer is presented with the opportunity to be taught.

TELEVISION'S IMPACT ON BEHAVIOR

Numerous theories have been developed to explain how television shapes perceptions and behaviors. Therefore, to make the argument that perceptions of HIV have been shaped by mediated narratives it is important to take a moment and understand how television educates audiences regardless of the intentions to do so. Central to many media theories, and one of the most widely investigated concepts, is involvement (Salmon 2001; Brown 2011). Brown argues that involvement, when broadly defined, is the degree of a person's psychological response to a mediated message. Thus, involvement should not be seen as a static or fixed idea. Rather, it is a dynamic process through which a viewer can become motivated both during and after media consumption (Rubin & Step 2000). While the majority of involvement research has focused on marketing and advertising studies, persuasion scholars have studied the various levels of a viewer's involvement with mediated messages and the connections between this involvement and motivation to alter one's behavior (Salmon, Witte, & Lee 2005; Murphy, Frank, Chatterjee, & Baezconde-Garbanati 2013). For example, if a viewer watches a character of a similar age, gender, and set of interests, they will be more likely to connect with the character. As a result of this new sense of connection, the viewer may begin to form parasocial, or one-sided, relationships with the character. Given the viewer's perception of similarity to and connection with the character, a viewer's involvement with a show or character may have a more powerful influence on their behavior than initially suspected (Hoffner & Buchanan 2005).

With the possibility for the development of parasocial relationships, one's involvement with a show or character, and the motivational functions this may have, becomes central to examining how involvement occurs. Research maintains that often viewers of health messages who have not personally experienced the topic at hand believe the myths provided by entertainment media as "secondhand reality" (Reese 2003, 9). The level of involvement with a show may explain the "reality" that is being created by the viewer. In other words, perception of HIV may stem from the way the topic is discussed by television shows.

Research has also found that viewers take more from shows they already like, or watch on a regular basis (Sparks 2015). Therefore, if a strong connection to a character results in the viewer being less likely to challenge the messages provided, the level of involvement may also be inherent (Murphy et al. 2011). The key to understanding involvement within these social models is to understand how the viewers are connecting with the show as well as how they resonate with the characters. While many public health theories have been used to examine and explain individuals' behaviors, two have directly spoken to how this notion of involvement with television serves as the motivation for behavior change.

Social Cognitive Theory

In an effort to explain how behaviors are modified, one of the most commonly applied theories in the area of E-E has remained Bandura's social cognitive theory (SCT). More specifically, SCT seeks to explain psychological functioning in terms of three determinants that continuously build upon and influence each other (Bandura 2001). First are the personal determinants, which form cognitive and affective conceptions of events around us. People are thought to be self-organizing, self-reflecting, and self-regulating organisms, thus personal determinants are directly impacted by two additional determinants: behavioral and environmental experiences. Overall the theory explains that cognitive factors, drawn from personal experiences, partly determine which environmental events will be observed as well as the meaning that individuals place upon them. Ultimately these constructions serve as the motivations and rationalizations for final behavior outcomes.

Overall SCT has been used extensively to explain health behaviors. In terms of HIV prevention, existing literature has supported the utility of social cognitive theory (DiIorio, Dudley, Soet, Watkins, & Maibach 2000). Previous research has examined a wide variety of topics ranging from the use of targeted interventions to increase female prisoners' efficacy in taking preventative measures (Exner, Seal, & Ehrhardt 1997) to college student use of condoms (Caron, Davis, Halteman, & Stickle 1993; Sheeran, Abraham, & Orbell 1999), even the use of radio programs to disprove commonly held HIV myths in third world countries (Rogers et al. 1999).

By observing others who appear to be similar, viewers can learn vicariously by witnessing the interactions and consequences of those they observe (Bandura 2001). Social models, such as those on television, are thought to transmit "knowledge, values, cognitive skills, and new styles of behavior" to viewers (Bandura 2004, 78). Bandura argues that for the translation of health knowledge into effective preventative behaviors to occur, social and self-regulative skills and a sense of personal power to exercise control over sexual and drug activities must be present. As health topics continue to be present within meditated narratives, the promotion of behavioral change can be achieved by informing, enabling, motivating, and guiding the audience (Bandura 2004).

It should be noted, however, that one important caveat to SCT is that not all observed behaviors are imitated (Moyer-Guse 2008). In particular, Moyer-Guse notes that SCT contains "four cognitive sub processes that govern observational learning, including attention, retention, production, and motivation" (412). Moyer-Guse argues that this final process, motivation, is a key part of the theory, and accounts for the fact that people do not choose to engage in every behavior they learn (Bandura 1986). Rather, an individual must be motivated to enact the behavior. As such, motivation appears to be influenced by outcome expectancies and self-efficacy (Moyer-Guse 2008).

Outcome expectancies refers to the observer's perceptions of the consequences (positive and/or negative) that are likely to result from a given behavior. Observing a character in a show that is rewarded for his or her behavior can serve to positively motivate and reinforce the behavior in the mind of the viewer. In the case of sexual behaviors, this could take the form of continuing to show characters engaging in risky behaviors, such as unprotected sex, with no illustration of consequences. On the other hand, when behaviors are modeled through characters being punished or shown becoming pregnant or contracting an STI, negatively reinforced outcomes are presented (Bandura 2004). Overall, for learning through observation to occur the social models and characters presented must frame the messages in a way that encourages involvement and decreases counter-arguing.

Extended Elaboration Likelihood Model

While it is common for SCT to be included in E-E studies, recent theorizing about narrative persuasion in entertainment-education has also included the Extended Elaboration Likelihood Model (E-ELM) (Slater & Rouner 2002). This model focuses its attention on the unique ability of E-E to influence beliefs, attitudes, and behavior by reducing viewers desires to argue with the messages presented (Slater & Rouner 2002). Specifically, E-ELM states that when viewers are engaged in an entertainment aspect of a television show they are less likely to be critical of the messages presented (Morgan & Shanahan 2010). Moreover, the deeper the viewer is engaged in the medium the greater the influence these frames will have on beliefs, attitudes, and behaviors. This theory also discusses two main components of engagement, including transportation and identification with characters.

Transportation

According to the theory of transportation, viewers of television can become completely immersed in a story, leaving the real world behind (Green, Brock, & Kaufman 2004; Valkenburg & Peter 2013). Brown (2011) notes that the theory of transportation particularly describes the process of how audiences are emotionally and psychologically transported into a media. Brown argues that the more viewers observe a character the greater connection they feel to them, regardless of the show being perceived as real or fictional. It is this connection, and liking of a character, that leads to selective exposure to certain media personas (Zillmann & Bryant 1985). Through this process, audience members develop an emotional and psychological connection with the characters, at times to the extent that they imagine themselves in the show.

Vital to the notion of transportation is its ability to reduce counter-arguing, given that viewers are swept up in the narrative and thus not motivated to challenge the stories' messages (Green & Brock, 2000; Knowles & Linn, 2004; Slater & Rounder, 2002). Empirical evidence has supported the idea that transportation into a narrative can increase acceptance of the messages contained in a narrative, even after controlling for initial attitudes several weeks earlier (Green & Brock 2000; Murphy, Frank, Moran, & Patnoe-Woodley 2011). By including a narrative about HIV into a television program consistently followed by the target population, the impact of the message could be increased.

Examining one's transportation into a show offers an integral understanding of how television echoes real-life dramas, and how it serves to reinforce credibility by presenting familiar and true-to-life stories that appeal to viewers' interests (O'Donnell 2016). Yet for these narratives to be effective, they also must be accessible, easily understood, fall within the range of plausibility, and strike viewers as familiar enough to be relatable (Madhu, Malan, Engebretsen, Hashmi, Sharma, & Etzenhouser 2009). To achieve this goal, the characters and storylines used must be presented in a way that viewers identify similarities.

Identification

Identification refers to the emotional and cognitive process of a viewer forgetting about his or her own reality and temporarily becoming the character, taking on the character's perspective (Cohen 2001). During this process the viewer shares in the experience and imagines what it would be like to be the character. This imagining "replaces his or her personal identity and role as audience member with the identity and role of the character" (251). This process is thought to occur on four varying dimensions: empathic (shared feelings with the character), cognitive (sharing the character's perspective), motivational (internalizing the character's goals), and absorption (the loss of self-awareness during exposure) (Cohen 2001).

As Moyer-Guse (2015) points out that in many ways identification and transportation can be observed as similar. Noting that the fourth dimension in the definition of identification, absorption, overlaps with the definition of transportation. However, it can also be argued that identification goes beyond transportation into a show. Identification must also take into consideration the other dimensions directed at one particular character within the narrative rather than just a storyline overall.

Identification also occurs when an individual adopts the attitudes, values, or beliefs of another individual or group based on a "self-defining" relationship (Kelman 1961, 63). Thus perceived similarities occur when an individual perceives that he or she is similar to a character. These similarities may refer to physical attributes, demographic variables, beliefs, personality, or values (Eyal 2004). In effect, each of these areas of similarity aid in the connection a viewer may experience with a character, increasing the likelihood of a viewer to identify with and become involved with the show (Moyer-Gusé, Chung, & Jain 2011).

The study of identification as a process of social influence is especially applicable to studying involvement with media characters, because people regularly identify with the characters they see on television and are often influenced by the messages with which they are presented (Hoffner & Buchanan 2005). As such, identification can arguably be understood as a process of social change in which an individual who has established a relationship with a character on a show allows the character's attitudes, values, beliefs, and behavior to influence the viewer, resulting in the reinforcement of existing attitudes, values, beliefs, and behavior perceived to be similar to those of the persona or the adoption of new ones modeled by the character (Brown 2011).

Theory of Entertainment Persuasion

Identifying that more work was needed to understand how E-E functioned persuasively, Moyer-Guse (2008) combined elements of two leading theories, SCT and the E-ELM. Looking specifically at the areas of transportation and identification, she postulates that the higher the level of transportation results in the decreased likelihood of counterargument with the message presented. Examining the involvement with narrative storylines and characters that is fostered by entertainment programming, Moyer-Guse offers an explanation and separation of several related constructs, such as identification, parasocial interaction, similarity, and others. Overall, she argues that the more a viewer connects to the characters of a show, due to perceived similarity, they will accordingly have an increased level of perceived vulnerability. In other words if a viewer feels connected to a character, and sees that character concerned about sexual health, the viewer may be more likely to become concerned about their own behaviors.

Motivating Change through Entertainment Education

Exposure to health information in popular programs has been found to not only increase knowledge, but also significantly increase attitudes and a person's desire to engage in preventative behaviors (Murphy et al. 2011). Researchers believe E-E influences the external environment of the audience. This influence is then vital to creating the necessary conditions for social and system level changes to occur. If audiences are under the impression that an issue, such as HIV, is no longer important, then one would not be expected to make attempts to increase prevention measures. However, as discussed throughout this chapter, talking about an issue and raising the awareness of the general population, not only could the perception of susceptibility increase but so too could the understanding of the need for policy or structural change. As a result, E-E can function as a social mobilizer, advocate, and agenda setter, influencing public and policy initiatives in a socially desirable direction (Wallack, Dorfman, Jernigan, & Themba 1993).

One way social mobilization occurs is through the way an issue is discussed, or framed by the media. Specifically, one of the largest concerns for E-E scholars is the use of negative frames. In these cases the frames used appear to define the issue at hand in a negative way as to encourage only certain interpretations and to discourage others (Goffman 1974). In many ways the frames used by television media profoundly influence audience perception, hence functioning as a means of social construction. However, it is here that E-E practitioners and scholars alike must pay the closest attention. According to the theory of social representation, individuals gather information about an inexperienced or unknown phenomena and will examine media's representation as the first step, and build their own frame of public opinion from these representations (Murphy 2007). As a result, television media becomes crucial for increasing, or decreasing, a viewer's understanding of their own susceptibility and the severity of a health issue.

Driving any behavioral change, a perception of severity and awareness of susceptibility must be present. In other words, if a person a.) regards himself as susceptible to a condition, b.) believes this condition will lead to serious consequences, c.) believes that a change in behaviors will lead to the lowering of the susceptibility or severity of the condition, while d.) also believing these actions to be of greater benefit than the original behaviors, *then* modification of behaviors will occur. Extensively studying how people change behavior, across a wide variety of actions and contexts, Prochaska and DiClemente (1992) developed the transtheoretical model of behavior change (TTM), finding that people go through a series of stages when changing behavior. These researchers view the stages more as a continuum of motivational readiness than rigid steps toward changing behavior. Progressing along the change continuum is an important aspect of a successful intervention, even if it does not immediately produce the desired behavioral change. However, before any movement is expected, the individual must feel a desire, or need, to change the behavior. Given the prevalence of sex in the media it might be assumed that multiple opportunities have been presented to raise awareness about safer sexual health behaviors, unfortunately this has not been the case.

MOTIVATING SEXUAL HEALTH BEHAVIORS THROUGH ENTERTAINMENT EDUCATION

Over the years, studies such as these have supported the conclusion that the amount of sexual content on TV has been increasing considerably over the years (Greenberg & Woods 1999; Bleakley, Hennessy, & Fishbein 2009). In fact, the percentage of TV programs containing sexual content has significantly risen from 56 percent in the 1997–98 television season to 70 percent of shows in 2004–05 (Kunkel et al. 2005). More recently, slightly more than 1 in 10 programs (11%) have included some form of sexual intercourse portrayals (Ward, Reed, Trinh, & Foust 2014). Due to censorship, most programs rarely show explicit portrayals of sexual intercourse. However, producers have found many creative ways of implying sexual activity including the use of sexual noises or visuals (eg., cars rocking or steaming windows) within a scene, or showing a couple entering or leaving a bedroom hand in hand. In terms of the percentage of shows containing sexual behaviors, nearly 75 percent of prime time shows contained some form or mention of sexual content with only 14 percent of the sexual incidents mentioning any risk or consequence for such activities. Risks associated with sexual activity (e.g., contraction of an STI or unplanned pregnancy) have been seldom included as themes in television (Gunasekera et al. 2005).

While many of the actual sexual encounters portrayed on television may be merely implied rather than explicitly shown, they have still been found to have a profound impact on viewers (Boot, Peter, & van Oosten 2014). To gain insight into how these messages are affecting audiences, scholars have conducted a great deal of research examining the proliferation of sexual content in the media. Focusing on college students' viewing of reality television, which is known for higher levels of sexual content, research has revealed that those who consistently viewed shows such as *16 and Pregnant* (Aubrey, Behm-Morawitz, & Kim 2014), *Temptation Island*, or *The Real World* (Zurbriggen & Morgan 2006) were not only more likely to share a sexual double standard in terms of the roles of men and women but were also more inclined to engage in riskier sexual behaviors. As a result, scholars continue to argue that exposure to sexual content in entertainment programming can contribute to a young person's sexual socialization (Sutton, Brown, Wilson, & Klein 2001; Brown et al. 2006).

With many of the United States' sex education programs choosing to remain focused dominantly on abstinence-only programs, the media has arguably become the leading source of sexual education for young viewers (Strasburger, Wilson, & Jordan 2009). However, the United States is also ranked as having of the most sexually suggestive media in the world (Strasburger, Wilson, & Jordan 2009), using sex to sell anything from cars to movie tickets. As a result, viewers receive a multitude of mixed messages, with most working against effective safe sex education. Scholars have compared the American media's use of sex to a harmless sport, one which requires little to no protection, everyone can and should engage in, and has few consequences to be seen (Ferris, Smith, Greenberg, & Smith 2007; Strasburger, Wilson, & Jordan 2009; Kelly & Smith 2006).

Only a dozen or so studies have examined the relationship between the amount of sexual content viewed on TV and early onset of sexual intercourse (Ward & Friedman 2006). Specially, some studies have revealed that black female teenagers' exposure to rap music videos or X-rated movies is associated with the likelihood of multiple sexual partners or testing positive for an STI (Wingood, DiClemente, Harrington, Davies, Hook, & Oh 2001). In contrast, teenagers whose parents control their TV-viewing habits are less sexually experienced (Fisher, Hill, Grube, Bersamin, Walker, & Gruber

2009; Wright 2011). Finally, exposure to sexual content in the media can play a significant factor in the intention to have sex in the near future (Primack, Douglas, Fine, & Dalton 2009; Ward, Reed, Trinh, & Foust 2014). As noted by Eyal and Finnerty (2007), much of the previous research has indicated that outcomes of intercourse experienced by characters on television can indeed affect viewers. For example, they note, "among emerging adults, viewing television dramas that displayed negative emotional consequences for intercourse (e.g., feeling guilt) led to more negative attitudes toward premarital sex as compared with pre-exposure attitudes" (149).

Overall, the research on the influence of exposure to televised sexual consequences helps contribute to the growing body of evidence regarding the effects of exposure to sexual content on television (e.g., Aubrey et al. 2003; Collins et al. 2003; Pardun et al. 2005; Taylor, Alexopoulos, & Ghaznavi 2016) and specifically the portrayal of sexual intercourse on a variety of sexual attitudes and perceptions (Aubrey & Smith 2016; Farrar 2006; Taylor 2005). Thus, these studies as well as others offer support for the argument that television is still the dominant source of sexual socialization information (Rideout, Roberts, & Foehr 2005; Scull, Malik, & Kupersmidt 2014).

With sex remaining a dominate theme on nearly every channel and young adults immersing themselves in large quantities of television viewing, the potential for the messages presented to impact the way viewers perceive sex and consequences for risky behaviors is virtually guaranteed. As mentioned previously, the majority of the extant research done in this area has focused on content analyses, providing a discussion of how sexual content is presented on television. Such research has offered understanding of television's portrayal of sexual intercourse and its outcomes. Specifically, research has found topics such as HIV and STIs in shows often affect perceptions of the meaning and act of sex as well as the development and maintenance within relationships (Galincian 2004) and understandings of one's own sexuality (Eyal 2010), as well as the means of talking about sex to peers and partners (Kim, Sorsoli, Collins, Zylbergold, Schooler, & Tolman 2007).

Gilk et al. (1998) argue that often a show's ability to make an impact will depend on content as well as the context of message. As a result, Gilk and colleagues provide a challenge for researchers to examine the rhetorical functions of E-E. By examining these rhetorical functions, the initial phase of study seeks to uncover possible areas where miseducation could be occurring. Considering that research has consistently found that television can dramatize everyday social problems, it becomes vital to examine the ways that these mediated HIV narratives perpetuate or challenge current perceptions regarding sexual health and behavior. Therefore, the following chapter offers a deeper look at the various meanings and contexts in which HIV has been discussed while also offering insight into how one can critically examine mediated messages.

Chapter Two

Conceptualizing HIV in the Media

Television narratives provide a variety of messages and meanings. Thus, as a viewer, one must be attentive to every possible layer. Polysemy, or possibility for a message to carry multiple meanings, of televised narratives therefore offers rich texts for examination. Taking on the role of a television critic allows for a viewer to not only combat misinformation and fear mongering, but also redistributes power. Although many viewers might prefer to remain focused on the entertainment and simple enjoyment provided by television, the ability to critically analyze mediated narratives accurately enables a fuller and richer understanding (Biesecker 1989). Seeking to provide you with the tools needed for such an endeavor, this chapter is organized around some of the key components of television criticism. The primary concern here is to explain the approaches used to examine HIV narratives, as well as explaining the merits for doing so.

CONTEXTS WITHIN TELEVISION

One of the most critical aspects of communication is context. Nothing occurs in a vacuum; therefore, the setting, background, characters, and motivations are each incredibly important. This context is not only true for the issue of how HIV has been presented on television but also for this chapter. Thus, the first goal is to introduce the large and complicated context surrounding HIV. Before the analysis of HIV narratives can begin it must be clear why these narratives are important. Beyond setting the initial stage, it should also be understood that similar to the choices we have in watching one show over another, many specific and critical choices were made in the process of writing this book. These choices are for two reasons. First, these choices should help understand the why and how this study was accomplished. Such choices will be vital when exploring how the media has framed an issue over time.

While teaching my own students I am always seeking models they can follow, thus the goal is that this book may serve that purpose for others. Second, and possibly even more importantly, is the goal to awaken the ability to challenge what is seen in the media. As consumers of media it is imperative that we consider the messages taken in. As I will discuss in chapter two, even without thinking about it, and advertisers hope you are not, we absorb hundreds of messages every day. From what to wear, eat, do for fun, and how to behave, the media shapes our understanding of a wide variety of topics. For the current and future writers and producers of the media, I want to make it clear that we must be more diligent about how health topics are presented. Therefore, let me begin by talking briefly about why *how* we talk about health is important.

THE HIV SITUATION

My particular concern with HIV discourse on television centers on the impact such conversations have. From a rhetorical standpoint, the way we talk about an event, social problem, or even a natural disaster frames what we know and perceive. Such discourses are argued to either originate as a response to the event (also known as the *exigence*), or help in the shaping of the situations themselves (Biesecker, 1989). In the case of HIV, I argue the rhetorical situation is largely both. Given the manner through which HIV is transmitted,[1] and the pandemic levels of infections, the conversation is undeniably warranted. Messages about the HIV transmission, prevention, and awareness of medical advancements each constitute discourse. However, part of what has prolonged the HIV situation we know today, is the way HIV has been and continues to be discussed.

Unlike many illnesses, HIV is almost always acquired as a result of precarious behaviors. Therefore, many people feel justified in saying that HIV is a punishment for poor choices. Such a mindset can then be used to support stigma, fear, and lack of compassion. While overt expressions of stigma, including banning people living with HIV from schools, places of work, and restaurants, have decreased over the years, inaccurate beliefs about the risks posed by casual social contact still remain.

From a public health perspective, what is even more concerning is the number of people who will not seek testing given the fear of being judged, or assumed to be in anyway connected to "those types of people." When media chooses to only focus on certain behaviors, and populations, viewers quickly learn who will receive the punishment of HIV. As a result, many people, engaging in risky behaviors, still refuse to obtain necessary testing.

What's Holding Us Back?

Looking at any rhetorical situation *constraints* of the situation must be taken into consideration. Constraints are barriers, or obstacles, that may be shaping the discourse. For HIV, three primary constraints are in play. First is the issue that talking about sexual behavior remains widely accepted as a taboo topic in the United States. While sex is prevalent across every platform of popular culture, when it comes to speaking about behaviors and/or sexual health, the lines of communication shut down. Characters are shown in nearly every stage of sexual activity all hours of the day, but in comparison televised activities or conversations include condoms, testing, or STIs in general. However, when an episode of *Friends* included a direct and poignant discussion about the effectiveness of condoms, ratings soared and scholars found that viewers were able to identify the episode as prompting the need for sexual health discussions (Collins, Elliott, Berry, Kanouse, & Hunter 2003).

Why HIV, STIs, and sexual health are considered taboo topics is in large part due to the second constraint: religious viewpoints. Many of the dominant religions value sexual behavior as a sacred activity for married partners, for the purpose of procreation. In his book, *Forbidden Fruit: Sex & Religion in the Lives of American Teenagers,* Mark Regnerus (2007) discusses how the culture in America has remained deeply limited in openness when discussing sexuality, especially the activities of young adults. Everything from purity pledges to the ways in which religious tenants create uneasiness or guilt. Ultimately, however, Regnerus finds young adults rarely state that religion has prevented them from engaging in sexual activity.

Discussions of sexual health have also been shaped by the political influences on sex health education. Regardless of a school being religious, private, or public the dominant narrative for decades has been "just don't have sex." Shifting away from comprehensive health programs, many schools argued abstinence education discourages teenage sexual frequency and onset by increasing the perceived cost of having sex, leading to a lower incidence of teen pregnancy and STIs (Carr & Packham 2016). Conversely, research has adamantly shown that abstinence-based programs do not work. In fact, Carr and Packham found that from 2000–2011 state-level abstinence education mandates had no effect on teen birth rates or abortion rates. Additionally, many schools' "time in the classroom" continues to be dictated by the need to prepare students for standardized tests, and given that sexual health education is not included on such tests, many schools having the option to include sex education in their curriculum choose not to.

Due to the possible combinations of each of these constraints it must be noted that television is not the only place where a lack of conversation about HIV in the United States is occurring. Scholarship of HIV narratives has dominantly focused on every other country around the world. From HIV-positive puppets in Africa[2] to the wealth of characters discussing HIV within telenovelas, scholars have spent a significant amount of time examining how HIV is presented in the media of other places. Minimal amounts of research have been conducted examining the narratives here at home. To date only three books have examined HIV in the media, one of which focused only limitedly on the United States. Yet even the most current is already sixteen years old. Thus, a primary purpose of this book is to relaunch the conversation. What are we teaching via mediated narratives here in the United States? To start this conversation, a few important decisions had to be made.

DIFFICULT CONVERSATION, DIFFICULT CHOICES

As a qualitative and rhetorical scholar, the majority of my research has involved an inductive approach. In other words, vast amounts of data and texts are examined by looking for connections, themes, and arguments. It is fascinating how the texts themselves provide multiple meanings. Providing each viewer of a show, or reader of a text, the ability to see/hear something that stands out for them. Be sure to understand, a "text" is not limited to the literal words on a page. Rhetorical texts, or artifacts, come in many forms; in the case of this book the episodes of each show provide a unique text for analysis.

Choices in which meanings to narrow in on impacts the arguments presented. In the process of conducting the present research, numerous choices were made. Each choice provides a specific lens through which the texts are examined. These choices also mean that other lenses are not being used, and therefore careful consideration and justification must be provided. For starters, throughout the process of collecting shows containing an HIV narrative, two primary considerations were taken. First was the choice to focus on shows aired in the United States. The focus of the present research is how people in the United States perceive risk of HIV, therefore for the current project, shows aired in other countries are only included as a specific point of comparison. However, additional work is underway comparing the HIV narratives across countries. The second consideration was the popularity of a show. Databases, online queries, and previous research was utilized to generate the list of shows for analysis. Over sixty different shows and made-for-TV movies were identified as continuing at least one episode where HIV was a primary plotline. Of which 15 shows provided multiple episodes, four including an entire season.[3] However, on a few occasions a show was found to only briefly mention HIV, thus did not create a larger storyline surrounding the topic; in these instances the episode would not be included for analysis. Once collected each show was reviewed, transcribed, and analyzed.

The HIV Genre

Not all shows are created equal when it comes to teaching viewers about HIV. Structurally some programs lend themselves better to in-depth conversations about life and death issues. Viewers of a drama expect heart strings to be pulled, and would not be shocked to see a character struggle, even die. Conversely, viewers of comedy seek to be lifted up, made to laugh, and would only expect to see a character perish in a funny, piano from the sky, kind of way. In other words, the genre of a show impacts not only what is said in the show but also who the audience might include.

Considering genres and subgenres of a show aids in understanding how a story will be told. Every genre will share similar characteristics and features. This use of similar features allows new audience members to join in on a show already in progress. Although the new viewer might not know the history between two characters, the dynamics between characters in love, or two nemeses, often look similar across shows. For example, within a dramatic genre tension is created for the audience through conflict. The type of conflict found in the drama is then used to create smaller categories, or subgenres. One such subgenre is the crime or legal drama. In these shows character development is centrally based on themes involving criminals (the antagonists), law enforcement, and the legal system (often serving as protagonist).

Although HIV narratives have appeared in a variety of genres the topic has been found most consistently in the areas of news, drama, and comedy. Not only have HIV and AIDS been repeatedly covered within each of these genres but also across multiple subgenres (including medical dramas, crime dramas, teen dramas, situational comedy, animated comedy, and standup comedy). Further discussion of the formatting and subgenres is provided in chapters four and five. Although drama and comedy genres have their own unique characteristics, basic structural components provide points for analysis.

The Structure of HIV

Understanding that people often learn through the observation of others (Bandura 2001) it is vital to understand what people are seeing. What characters are shown talking about, living with, and dying of HIV on television? How is the topic of HIV being brought into the shows themselves? What medical information is presented, if any? Each of these questions can be examined by evaluating the narrative structures of an episode where HIV is discussed. Thus, the second choice made for this book was to examine how HIV was shown on television over the course of the virus, thus the use of structural criticism.

Structural criticism guides the analysis of how a narrative is constructed. Conducting structural criticism of mediated HIV narratives means that not only examining the use of HIV in the plotline of the narrative, but also looking across the stories, and shows, comparing the evolution of the storyline over time. The following table breaks down specifically how each show was structurally examined.

SUMMARY

To better understand where stigma, fear, and lack of behaviors change might stem from, this book examines over three decades of HIV narratives presented in prime-time television. Beginning with the first televised narrative of the mysterious "gay cancer," HIV from conception has created a rhetorical situation ripe for examination. My goal is to provide understanding of the many levels one must consider when examining mediated discourse. This chapter presented an argument for why we should consider how HIV is discussed on television, and provided a brief look into why HIV remains a taboo topic for conversation and analysis. Additionally, this chapter introduces genres and

Table 2.1. Breakdown of Structural Criticism Framework.

Character	Characters with HIV (or who thought they were at risk) were each analyzed by: HIV status, race, age, sexual orientation, occupation, whether the character died from HIV.
Plot	How the topic of HIV was brought into the show's story. Questions asked about each plotline included: Was the HIV storyline central to the episode or a secondary focus; was the plotline completed in one show, or across multiple episodes; what types of conflict were included within the plotline?
Tone	Tone commonly includes music, lighting, pace of the dialogue. Even more important for this analysis was the way characters talk to each other and about HIV. Where characters were shown given support, judged, discriminated against, etc.
Medical Accuracy	Although not a typical structural comment for narrative analysis, when a show includes a major health topic the ability for accurate information to be shown is key. Therefore, facts about HIV, discussion of common HIV myths, and testing being shown or mentioned was carefully considered.

The table provides insight into how each episode was examined from a structural perspective.

structural components used to conduct the research discussed in part two of this book.

To illustrate specifically how HIV narratives have functioned as educational tools, part two critically examines three specific genres of television where the mixture of education and entertainment can be observed. These chapters investigate how each genre has presented facts and other educational information about HIV, regardless of their intent to do so. Additionally, the following section examines how narrative structures, such as the structure of the show, characters and situations/themes used to introduce the topic, as well as the conclusions or ramifications presented within a show, impact viewers' perceptions of their own risk for HIV.

NOTES

1. Only certain body fluids—blood, semen, pre-seminal fluid, rectal fluids, vaginal fluids, and breast milk—from a person who has HIV can transmit HIV. When these fluids come in contact with a mucous membrane, or damaged tissue, or are directly injected into the bloodstream (from a needle or syringe), transmission can occur. Mucous membranes are found inside the rectum, vagina, penis, and mouth.
2. The South African version of the children's educational program *Sesame Street* has introduced an HIV-positive character. The program, aimed at very young children, wants to show that those living with HIV are no different to others and should be treated as such.
3. See Appendix A for a list of all shows included in the analysis.

2

Previously On . . . HIV on Television

Chapter Three

This Just In, HIV in the News

It is said that news channels don't tell viewers what to think, but instead what to think about. In essence networks serve as a viewer's neck, turning their head in the direction the media sees fit. Suggesting that news media is vital to the start of any discussion, as well as setting the agenda for the discussion, mass media scholars McCombs and Shaw (1972) developed the agenda-setting function theory. They argue that everyone involved in news production, from editors to broadcasters, have a hand in shaping an audience's sense of reality. Essentially, one's reality is shaped by the series of issues and stories media producers have chosen to cover frequently and prominently. Thus, turning the head of the audience, persuading audiences to regard the issue as important. Reflecting on what will make the head turn, American journalist, Armstrong Williams has been quoted saying, "There are two sayings that are familiar in every news room across the country: 1) sex sells; 2) if it bleeds it leads." That is unless the "blood" is the result of sexual, or drug related, behaviors.

Although the first case of what is now known as HIV was documented in the United States in the late 1960s, it was not until 1981 that the "illness" made its media debut in an article in *The Los Angeles Times* (Kinsella 1989). Starting off as an abstract discussion of the mysterious "gay cancer" the discourse surrounding HIV eventually found it's human frame in the 1990s. About a decade later HIV narratives worked their way into nearly every aspect of political and popular culture. The messages produced by news networks not only shaped the way viewers learned the "facts" of HIV, but they also played a major role in shaping the messages echoed within popular television shows. To understand media's contribution to the education and miseducation of viewers we must start with the messages and the frames of those messages. Examining archived evening news reports and previous research on how HIV has been covered by major new outlets, this chapter offers an overview of 35 years of HIV coverage.

FRAMING HIV/AIDS

Undoubtedly, all major news platforms have their own agendas for what is considered news. Fox News is known for its conservative framing, while CNN is (often) labeled as a liberal news source. The notion of framing comes from the work of sociologist Erving Goffman (2009). Within much of Goffman's work he argues that media focuses an audience's attention on certain events, thus placing them within a field of meaning. In the case of HIV, over three decades of content and framing seem to have been shared across every platform. Meaning that regardless of the typical lens used by news outlets, the coverage overall shared similar viewpoints. As if reading from a communal playbook, from the beginning of the epidemic, networks shared experts and interpretations, disseminating the same fears and narrow views. Consequently, news outlets have not only held the power to raise awareness of HIV, they have also shaped the opinions and understandings of the virus.

The Abstract 80s

Even with thousands of people dying of a "mysterious illness," it is rare that severity of an issue alone will raise the attention of media gatekeepers, those who will decide the newsworthiness of a topic. In the early 1980s the CDC and other medical groups had published articles and reports about what would later become known as HIV, the virus that causes AIDS. Yet most of what was covered, even after mainstream news outlets jumped on board, presented a vague, fear-driven medical frame.

Men in white coats explained, "We have a new disease here. It was not here ten years ago, and we have no cure." Without a specific name for the illness abstract phrases such as "mysterious cancer," "new deadly STD," "serious public health problem" were repeated sound bites. Two major consequences resulted from the sterile and abstract discussions: mass panic and fear. Given the amount of time it took to gain the media's attention about the illness, hundreds of people had already died, and thousands more would die within the next few years. With nearly every person who presented symptoms dying, it was only logical that headlines and news stories would use words such as "deadly," "killer," and "crisis." Thus, fear of death from the unknown killer plagued the nation.

News audiences at this time were also confused about how the illness was acquired. Admittedly, little was known at first about how the "mysterious cancer" was contracted, therefore people were quick to become fearful of anything others might have come in contact with, including everything from doorknobs to toilet seats. After emergency rooms and doctor's offices became flooded with questions and worries, researchers from the CDC came forward announcing the illness was not acquired through breathing the same air of others, that no hospital workers had contracted the disease, and that the only way to contract the virus was through contact with blood or semen. However, squeamish journalists continued to describe the mode as "an exchange of fluids." Leaving "fluids" open to interpretation, fluids mistakenly included saliva, tears, and mist expelled from sneezing or coughing.

Not only were people fearful, due to the severity of the illness, but fear was also induced given the uncertainty of who was as risk. Initial reports stated the illness was "primarily" being seen in gay populations. Thus, one of the initial names for the illness was GRID (gay-related immune deficiency). Without specifics of how GRID was transmitted, the second consequence of the media's language became stigma toward anyone who could contract the illness.

From the beginning journalists struggled to find ways to discuss the issue of GRID. Reporters did not typically use words such as "anal intercourse" or "semen" on air. Additionally, producers even became concerned with how to describe the primary population being affected. Some editors, such as Ab Rosenthal the editor of *The New York Times,* insisted his reports use the medicalized label "homosexual" rather than "gay" (Kinsella 1989). While it is possible Rosenthal and others like him were unaware of the religious, legal, and medical underpinnings of the term "homosexual," the term had long been rejected, and deemed offensive, by the gay community. Equally, given the lack of understanding most people had about the gay community, connecting a deadly illness with the community only fueled a fire of stigma and fear.

In the next few years the knowledge of GRID would evolve and a new name would take it's place, AIDS (acquired immune deficiency syndrome). Yet, media outlets continued to focus on the issue regardless of the new name, and not the people AIDS was affecting. Positioning AIDS within one community and the "germ panic" created a perfect environment for moral panic and discrimination toward the "social deviants" (including homosexuality, promiscuity, and intravenous drug users) who would contract it. Media outlets focused attention on one or two specific cases, and not the numbers or trends found across the country. Thus, from the viewpoint of gay community, media outlets seemed to be trying to avoid drawing attention to the numbers of gay people dying.

It's wasn't until the mid-1980s that AIDS would be a primary focus within the media agenda. By 1985 all of the major news networks had begun airing AIDS-related stories on a regular basis. Within the first five years stories related to AIDS jumped from an average of 14 stories per month, to 143 stories per month (Singhal & Rogers 2003). Yet, regardless of the increase in coverage, journalists still framed the epidemic as an emergency, creating a sense of urgency by emphasizing dread, exaggeration, and fear.

With stories being generated daily, the frame of AIDS as a multilevel social problem was also presented. On an individual level people were afraid of how AIDS was transmitted. As a result, not only were citizens across the nation interviewed; medical providers—even police and firefighters—also reported a shared fear of AIDS. There were numerous cases where firefighters and emergency responders were quoted as being unwilling to help people in the gay community for fear of contracting AIDS. To combat the risk, first responders were given specialized masks to wear when resuscitating an individual, yet some continued to state they would refused if they knew the patient was gay.

Discrimination against the gay community in the name of "fear of contracting AIDS" played a significant role in news headlines and stories in the 80s. Cases of landlords evicting gay residents and bosses firing gay employees regardless of their AIDS status became commonplace. Interview after interview, roughly 65 percent of the stories examined included cases of men telling their tales of stigma and discrimination. Such stories often began with reporters highlighting how "gays have been described as a dangerous and violent group. One that corrupts children while infecting their communities with AIDS." Although time would prove that AIDS was not only a virus acquired within the gay community, years of media coverage may have instilled this idea for millions of viewers.

Media's framing of AIDS as a gay problem was quickly identified by religious groups as a punishment for immoral behaviors. Accusations of "knowingly sharing their tainted blood" or "engaging in immoral acts" were each followed by statements that "AIDS is God's vengeance on the homosexual population." Another issue with framing AIDS as a social, or gay, problem was that such a frame rarely captured the attention of government agencies. In one interview, a young man stated "This [AIDS] is not a political issue. It's not a medical issue. It's not a gay issue. It's a human issue. I don't want to die because of red tape." Unfortunately, thousands would die before the government would step in and organize efforts to better understand AIDS.

Eventually the government and lagging media outlets heard the call to get involved. Beloved actor Rock Hudson was discovered to have contracted AIDS. After Hudson's announcement Ryan White, a thirteen-year-old from Kokomo, Indiana, also made headlines, having contracted AIDS through a blood transfusion. Fighting for his right to attend school White's story quickly caught national attention and soon he joined Hudson as the faces of AIDS.

With new faces, the media's attention to AIDS increased tenfold. Focusing on these stories, AIDS made its way into the hearts and minds of millions of viewers including government officials and celebrities alike. For the first time since the illness began people reported in public opinion polls that AIDS was the number one social issue. In response, on October of 1987 President Reagan finally spoke out about AIDS, naming it "public enemy number one." Rallying the call, celebrities came out in droves, demanding funding for research and greater awareness. Leading the charge was co-star and once wife of Hudson, Elizabeth Taylor. Today, Taylor's foundation remains a dominant presence within awareness campaigns, support for those living with the virus, and policy change at local and global levels.

Ultimately, AIDS in the 80s is summed up by two words: silence and fear. Far too long media outlets remained silent about the raising epidemic. Silence from the media became so important that some reports indicate that journalists who dared to be the first to write or report on AIDS were fired and blacklisted from the journalism community (Singhal & Rogers 2003). Once the story broke, however, fear-driven reporting dominated, setting the tone that AIDS was a deadly killer attacking the gay community.

Although it might have been the gay community that was first affected, thousands of heterosexual individuals would soon also contract and die of AIDS. In a sense, the early 1980s can be classified as a time of pre-contemplation. The United States didn't know or simply wasn't worried about AIDS. Entering the mid- to late 80s a clear shift occurs, resulting in the new attention of celebrities speaking out. Consequently, shifting in the 1990s, media outlets and America's attention began to evolve to a state of contemplation. Finally, it became clear that media, government, and people alike have become directly focused on the susceptibility *and* severity of AIDS.

The Political 90s

By 1992, AIDS had become the leading cause of death for men in the United States between the ages of 25–44. Two years later, AIDS became the leading cause of death overall for all Americans in that age range. Of those living with the virus, more than half would be women. Although it was clear AIDS was indeed not a "gay disease" the vast majority of new reports still focused on, or at least mentioned, gay populations. Most never mentioned women at all. By 1999, it was impossible to ignore the pandemic that was HIV/AIDS, as cases increased worldwide to over 60 million people. As a result, HIV became an issue threaded throughout media outlets, government policies, research labs, and into homes.

Media gatekeepers were no longer concerned with the backlash from discussing a "gay disease." Instead, not reporting on AIDS meant a far greater loss of ratings and revenue. High-profile cases such as basketball star "Magic" Johnson and British music icon, lead singer of Queen, Freddie Mercury were just two of the many stars who played essential roles increasing awareness about HIV/AIDS. ACT UP protests across the country cried out for more HIV treatments, and the expansion of clinical trials for women and people of color. Feeding off the frenzy, media outlets played their part making it clear AIDS would remain the leading headline throughout the decade.

One headline, sparking the first of many governmental policies, was the death of Ryan White. Surprising his doctors, Ryan White lived five years longer than predicted. Dying in April 1990, one month before his high school graduation. Shortly following his death, Congress passed the Ryan White Comprehensive AIDS Resources Emergency (CARE) Act. CARE continues to work with local community-based organizations providing comprehensive systems of care including primary medical care and essential support services for people living with HIV who are uninsured or underinsured. Along with CARE, government funds were also distributed to researchers in hopes of finding a cure.

In 1994, new stories returned attention to the medical sides as researchers identified the first drug found to prevent the spread of HIV. Azidothymidine (AZT), an antiretroviral medication, reduced the replication of the virus and was found to lead to improvements in both symptoms and blood tests. Taken just twice a day as part of highly active antiretroviral therapy (HAART), AZT was combined with other drugs (known as "the triple cocktail"). Offering hope numerous reports stated that AZT was the much needed first step toward a cure, and that within a few years AIDS could be no more. Decades later, AZT did provide an encouraging step, but the cost and side effects left many people living with HIV untreated.

Beyond the hope of finding the cure for HIV, government programs also made headlines with each new system tasked with protecting those living with the virus. Early in the 1990s Congress enacted the Americans with Disabilities Act prohibiting discrimination against individuals with disabilities, including people living with HIV/AIDS. Shortly thereafter, Congress passed the AIDS Housing Opportunity Act, creating the Housing Opportunities for People with AIDS (HOPWA) program, provide housing assistance to people living with AIDS. Understanding the need for global unification UNAIDS, a joint United Nations program on HIV/AIDS began operations coordinating HIV/AIDS efforts in the 1996.

With significant attention on understanding, researching, and preventing HIV/AIDS it became impossible for people to ignore. Even within scholarly research, HIV/AIDS had become a leading topic regardless of the area of study. According to Palmgreen, Noar, Zimmerman, Edgar, and Freimuth (2008) by the end of the 1990s HIV/AIDS had become a normalized part of the American social and ecological context. Integrated into nearly every aspect of life, media's attention to AIDS had reached its pinnacle.

The Institutionalized 2000s

In 2002, UNAIDS reported that HIV/AIDS had become the leading cause of death in sub-Saharan Africa and the fourth biggest global killer. In response President George W. Bush created the United States President's Emergency Plan for AIDS Relief (PEPFAR). With new worldwide organizations and programs media sources also shifted focus from the number of HIV/AIDS cases at home to those in other parts of the world. As a result, news reports slowly declined in both the number as well as the amount of time discussing HIV/AIDS.

From 1993 up until roughly 2004 the number of stories and articles about HIV remained consistent. What changed was that headlines no longer reflected a focus on HIV or AIDS; instead the issue was buried within the message. It is not that HIV was no longer discussed, it had simply been absorbed into other issues. However, the same cannot be said today. Since 2010 the topic of HIV has almost entirely disappeared from the media.

Evolving from a mysterious illness to daily discussions, HIV/AIDS had become institutionalized into common culture. During the early 2000s, news coverage took a different and very dangerous turn. While in 1987 AIDS was seen as the number one issue facing Americans, by 2003 less than one percent of people reported feeling concerned (Palmgreen, Noar, Zimmerman, Edgar, and Friemuth 2008). With less people dying of AIDS, new medical treatments, and rapid testing coverage of HIV, created the false impression that AIDS was now all but cured. As a result, people nationwide entered into complacency, and eventually HIV fell into the background. Workplace policies and discrimination training, educational programs, countless public service announcements, and a multitude of community outreach efforts solidified HIVs place in popular culture but only as an undertone and not as a central issue. Between treatment, research, income support, and prevention the federal government had increased HIV/AIDS spending from $200,000 in 1981 to an estimated $6.3 billion in 2004 (Johnson & Coleman 2000). Beyond increased funding efforts at home numerous worldwide governmental organizations and programs were also created.

After nearly two decades of "AIDS talk," people developed compassion and AIDS fatigue (Kaiser Family Foundation 2006; Swain 2005). Audiences started to tune out messages, and editors no longer felt the topic was newsworthy (Brodie, Hamel, Kates, Altman, & Drew, 2004). Besides brief moments of breakthroughs, or "anniversary" events, nearly all information about HIV/AIDS beginning in the early 2000s came from medical organizations or celebrities.

SUMMARY

For the majority of the past 35 years the HIV/AIDS story has been told as a reaction to a variety of events: a "mysterious illness," protests for research, government finally stepping in, and the number of celebrities pushing the topic into media's attention. After each major event new reports would swell for a period of time, but soon declined until another event refreshed media interest. By 2010, only short and rare mentions of HIV are found. The ebb and flow could be justified as following what is newsworthy, or timely. However, other media outlets, including television writers, often look to what is trending in the news as inspiration. Thus, given that an average of 42,000 new infects per year continue for a preventable illness, this is not a topic that can be brushed aside.

Rhetorical scholar Loyd Bitzer argues that a rhetorical situation is developed as a response to a situation, which he calls exigence. In other words, the discourse surrounding an issue is sparked by the event, as seen in the new patterns presented in this chapter. However, Richard Vatz challenges this order, arguing it is the discourse that shapes a rhetorical situation. According to Vatz it is the rhetor, the speaker or writer, and not the situation that creates the meaning. Applying Vatz's framework it can then be argued that HIV is in part not seen as newsworthy because the conversations have been all but removed from the media. Without exposure to a consistent discourse, society feels justified in thinking that HIV is no longer an issue of concern.

Aside from the ebb and flow of reports on HIV and AIDS the themes found across the reports generally remained consistent. Journalistic and likely editorial decisions were made minimizing the severity of AIDS in the beginning. Early coverage tried to assuage public concern about AIDS in general, but due to the headlines and stereotypical images used, the framing of the AIDS crisis invoked deeply entrenched stigma and fear. By the mid-90s AIDS was mentioned in nearly 70 percent of stories (Swaine 2005). Over time however, coverage of HIV and AIDS has become less frequent, shorter, and often remains celebrity-driven.

With the exception of World AIDS Day, and other special events, HIV only makes headlines when a celebrity addresses the pubic, announcing they have contracted the virus. One such modern example occurred when Charlie Sheen exploded HIV across news and social media. Though much of the discourse focused on the lack of surprise, given Sheen's well-publicized exploits, the message that even straight men can contract the virus was clear. Sheen himself, in an interview with *Good Morning America,* spoke to the fact that HIV is rarely a topic people talk about anymore. With the country's attention back on the topic of HIV, updated facts on the numbers of people living with HIV, advances in medications, and prevention methods were quickly injected. These quick inoculations of HIV information might help increase awareness for those who are paying attention, however, the window is far too short. In no time at all the media had moved on to the next topic and HIV was placed back on its shelf.

Another manner through which celebrities grab the attention of the public is with the creation of countless public service announcements, shows, and movies. In the 80s and early 90s, the after school specials injected facts and warnings about the risks of unsafe sex and drug use. But viewers became accustomed, and frankly cynical, to the overt messaging television writers elected to imbed on HIV education inside daytime dramas, prime time programs, and even comedy specials. Similar to the news frames used to cover HIV, many of these programs chose themes that focused on medical facts and social deviants. Focusing on fictional dramas, the next chapters dissect HIV narratives by closely examining the variety of themes and plotlines used when talking about HIV and AIDS.

Chapter Four

Oh the Drama!

The Many Sides of HIV in Dramatic Shows

Television dramas are an ideal space for teaching through observation. Encompassing a range of interpersonal situations, dramatic narratives offer an audience a means for social comparison. Teaching views about themselves, how to interact (or not) with others, as well as providing opportunities to observe conversations about difficult topics. Spanning subgenres such as medical, criminal/legal, and teen drama, HIV and AIDS have been woven into over 30 dramatically themed US television shows (many spanning numerous episodes). Examining 35 years' worth of HIV and AIDS dramatic narratives, each episode has been transcribed, dissected, and scrutinized uncovering common themes (discussed here as well as in part three). Within an episode, a viewer can observe both internal and external conflict, learn moral lessons by seeing repercussions of actions, and sometimes gain a sense of hope when, just about, everything works out in the end. Specifically exploring the ways these narratives shape perceptions of risk, this chapter presents a critical review of the ways HIV has been presented across subgenres of drama. The chapter begins with an introduction to the structural components of drama. Diving into the shows themselves a discussion of the subgenres is presented offering a look specifically at the formatting of HIV in terms of situations, types of conflict, as well as discussing the important lessons found across plotlines and across decades.

THE DRAMATIC GENRE

Before examining the shows themselves, it is important to first unpack what it means for a show to be considered a drama. Although shows today commonly include a blend of dramatic and comedic elements, the classification of a show as a drama sets the viewer's expectations. For instance, all dramatic shows include basic narrative components such as variety in the cast of characters (including protagonists, villains, and sidekicks), some form of conflict (either internal, external, or environmental), and sequential timeline. These "rules" for a drama allow for a viewer to quickly understand what is happening in the show, even if episodes have been missed. Most dramatic shows run on a 60-minute time schedule to allow for the development of deeper, more involved plotlines to evolve. Thus, most episodes (even set within larger storylines) will follow a set-up, raise of conflict, climax, and resolution format. Ultimately, it is the structural format of the drama that plays a major role in how the viewer will engage with the story.

The first televised dramatic narrative of AIDS took place in NBC's 1985 made-for-TV movie *An Early Frost*. The movie focused on the life, and ultimately the death, of Michael Pierson, a thirtysomething white gay male played by Aidan Quinn. Michael, a Chicago attorney, contracts the virus after his longtime partner steps outside of the relationship with another man. Upon discovering his diagnosis, Michael returns home with the difficult challenge of breaking the news that he is not only homosexual, but that he also has AIDS. Over the course of film the central focus is on the emotional impact AIDS has on the family. Though it is clear the movie seeks to personalize what it is like to live with and die of AIDS, the primary narrative was between Michael and his father, who adamantly refuses to accept his son as a gay man.

As scholars (Hart 2014; Treichler 1999; Tulloch & Lupton 1997) have remarked, this film echoed society's current perspectives against the "AIDS body." Instead of attempting to rupture the stigma and fear surrounding those living with HIV and AIDS, *An Early Frost* simply repeated the common trope found in labeling and blaming those with the virus as "getting what they deserved" given their "immoral behaviors." Although *An Early Frost* was the first of its kind, writers and producers of subsequent dramas have, more commonly than not, replicated this frame.

Not even a year later, the topic of HIV and AIDS began appearing in other dramatic narratives, first occurring in soap operas and then across other weekly primetime shows. The move into these popular shows not only increased exposure to the message, given the loyal viewership of shows such as *ER*, *Law and Order*, or *Beverly Hills 90210*, but also the message could reach wider segments of people. Subgenres (including medical, legal/procedural, and family dramas) include heavy themes within a show centered around one context. Each format of the drama will dictate how HIV is brought into the narrative and ultimately the type of lesson potentially taught. Therefore, prior to examining specific components of narratives, such as the characters, settings, and structure (discussed in chapters six and seven), it is important to consider the types of narratives and how HIV and AIDS are written into drama.

Medical Dramas

The most expected context for an HIV plotline is a medical drama. Often taking place in a hospital or medical clinic these shows already include settings where conversations about illness, prevention, and treatment would be commonplace. Characters including medical providers and patients are already poised to have knowledge about the virus or to be shown affected by it. Viewers therefore are less likely to challenge the topic or information presented given the settings and context.

Of the seven medical dramas examined,[1] only two shows included HIV-positive doctors. In *St. Elsewhere*'s episode "Family Feud," (S4 E15) aired January 29, 1986, on NBC, Dr. Caldwell, played by Mark Harmon, is told of his AIDS[2] diagnoses after being attacked by a woman he had brought home from a bar. It is unclear if his AIDS was contracted by his past sexual encounters or the razor blade he was attacked with. Caldwell himself states, "You know I can't even count the number of women I've rolled in clover with. When I got lonely, I went looking. But when I found something it could have been a lot of people. Maybe I deserve this." Throughout the two episodes containing this storyline the tone remained dark and morose. While some discussion of treatments is included, the show focused more on the internal struggles with Caldwell's now limited life, "Right now I am trying to understand I have about 15 months to live. But I can't! It doesn't make sense. All my life I have been taught to win. There is no way the clock has run out." Speaking directly to the concerns that treatments at the time were limited, Dr. Caldwell states, "Antivirals are just popguns against AIDS. All you are doing is buying a few more sexless, sleepless nights." Regardless of the fact that Dr. Caldwell presented no symptoms of the virus he leaves his post at the St. Eligius hospital. Seasons later his former colleagues are informed of his death.

In juxtaposition to *St. Elsewhere*, NBC also introduced the second medical professional shown living with HIV in the 1999 season of *ER*: physician's assistant Jeanie Boulet played by Gloria Reuben. Breaking a number of HIV stereotypes, Jeanie was a straight African American doctor who remained a central figure on the show for many seasons. Extending the character past the typical "dealing with the diagnosis stage" allowed for the show to highlight the personal and professional drama someone living with

HIV would endure, including decisions about disclosure, treatment, and impact of working with a stigmatized illness. At first, Jeanie chose to manage her HIV alone, refusing to disclose her status to her employers, but when previous partner and colleague Dr. Peter Benton (played by Eriq La Salle) discovers her condition he attempts to have her banned from treating patients with open wounds. Jeanie's decision not to reveal her HIV status also resulted in having to seek treatment at another facility, and paying for the incredibly expensive medications out of pocket. Beyond the countless facts and realistic discussions of HIV, Reuben's character was one of the first to be shown living a fulfilling and long life with the virus. In fact years later, after having left the show in 2008, Jeanie reappeared in the fourteenth, and final, season of the show when her adoptive HIV-positive son was diagnosed with an unusual form of brain tumor. In the end, the role of Jeanie Boulet not only modeled for audiences the many complexities of HIV, but it also sparked a deep-seated fire for advocacy within Gloria Reuben.[3]

Shifting from the primary characters, when HIV comes into the story it can reasonably be assumed to occur as a patient conflict. In total, thirteen patients were admitted into the medical dramas with HIV-related stories. Topics such as abortion, mystery illnesses, and the need for kidney transplants were just some of the storylines used to bring HIV into the picture. Mirroring the times, most of the patients in the 80s and 90s were shown as gaunt and sickly, with many dying by the end of the episode. However, in addition to the ability for HIV-positive characters to walk out of the episode, as time and medical treatments advanced so too did the opportunity for more accurate information to be presented in the show. Unfortunately, only a few of the episodes took advantage of this opportunity.

The most controversial portrayal of HIV treatment was found in 1995 on CBS's *Chicago Hope*. In the episode an HIV-positive patient is told by his doctor (Vondie Curtis-Hall) of an experimental procedure where he would be injected with malaria,[4] "Basically, the malaria parasites jump-start the immune system into attacking the HIV cells" (*Chicago Hope*, S1 E16). When the patient agrees to undergo the malaria injections, the chief of staff's, Dr. Watters (Hector Elizondo), legal team intervenes. However, when the hospital's legal counsel (Peter Nichols) states that the hospital could look the other way if the patient is injected with malaria parasites, the treatment occurs. Though the patient is shown at the end of the episode shivering in his bed, it is three months later when the character is revisited and shown passing away of HIV regardless of the malariotherapy treatment. Upon airing the show medical providers began to speak out about the dangers presenting experimental treatments in primetime dramas.

> [It sends a] potentially dangerous message to the public in general and specifically to people who have AIDS or are HIV-positive," Bronston wrote of the

> episode's treatment of malariotherapy, which has been discredited by the Centers for Disease Control, the Food and Drug Administration and the World Health Organization. "I believe that *Chicago Hope* has unintentionally given incorrect information to AIDS patients and to the public, maybe even given them false hope."[5]

In response to Dr. Bronston's letter the *Chicago Hope* producers quickly reached out and brought Bronston on board as a consultant for future shows.

Another show seeking the advice of outside sources, this time the knowledge of the Kaiser Family Foundation, was ABC's *Grey's Anatomy*. A 2008 episode wove specific and accurate information about HIV transmission into a storyline about a pregnant HIV-infected woman. Although the episode did not directly emphasize stigma or fear related to being HIV-positive, the goal instead was to educate viewers about the ability of HIV-positive women to give birth to healthy HIV-negative babies, if they take the proper medication. Here, the viewer learns that not only is there a chance of having a healthy baby, but the doctor notes, "I wasn't telling you there is some chance your baby might not be born sick. I was telling you there is 98 percent chance your baby will be born perfectly healthy. A 98 percent chance. There is greater chance of your baby being born with Downs Syndrome then you passing your HIV to your child" (*Grey's Anatomy*, S4 E13). Yet, although this episode provides information about HIV, little else is discussed. Nothing is mentioned about how the mother-to-be contracted HIV or how she was "dealing with it" beyond her stating, "I was diagnosed at 19, and I have learned how to deal with it. However, I am not going to put that onto a baby. I am not going to bring a baby into this world knowing that he might possibly have this disease." It should be noted that, although this episode was one of the few that worked with an organization in its writing, the amount of time spent talking about HIV was the least of all the medical episodes examined. It also should be noted that, given the amount of times characters discuss or are shown engaging in sexual activity, there are many opportunities presented for safe sex or sexual health behaviors to be addressed; however, these topics are rarely mentioned.

Similar to the episode presented by *Grey's Anatomy*, a spinoff series, *Private Practice*, also does well in highlighting the possibility of living a long life with a diagnosis of HIV. But, just as *Grey's Anatomy* missed the opportunity to dispel popular misperceptions about the virus, so too did *Private Practice*. On two occasions the show makes attempts to tackle issues related to HIV. Interestingly, whereas one episode does an exceptional job incorporating the various methods of education, the other fails in a number of ways. The first of the episodes, titled "A Family Thing" (S1 E2), introduces a family with a very interesting problem: How do they tell their teenage son that he has been HIV-positive since he was a child? Wanting to avoid telling their son about the diagnosis until he turned 18, the parents could unfortunately wait no longer, given his recent interest in having sex. When the topic of sex initially is brought up by the young teen, Dr. Cooper immediately takes the moment to note "Condoms, lots of condoms. STDs [sexually transmitted diseases] don't care about the pill. Or better yet wait." In only a few lines the writers are able to get to the heart of the issue: the only way to keep protected from STDs is by condoms or abstinence.

Overall, this episode is distinctive for mentioning condoms first. Too often, when teenagers are shown talking about sex, the adult's primary focus is on abstinence only. Another advantage to this quick educational moment is the comment about STDs not caring about the pill. These words directly challenge the notion that condoms are only for pregnancy prevention. Thus, if interventions in this area seek to target the perceptions of condom use, televised messages will need to be considered as modes affecting health outcomes.

The episode also attempts to increase viewer perceptions of personal vulnerability or risk. This teen was diagnosed HIV-positive when he was five, but because his parents had yet to disclose this information to him, all he knew was that he had a kidney condition. This then communicates that anyone could be walking around not knowing he or she is HIV-positive and, therefore, regular testing is essential. His parents argued that they were protecting him from stigma and discrimination. In hindsight, however, their "protection" was only blinding their son to the truth, which means a higher chance of infecting others. The writers of the television show present an effective way of targeting this particular subject. However, the average viewer may not pick up on this controversial subject because it is not advanced directly. Overall, this episode is effective in engaging the viewer. Presenting HIV not only as something that anyone, even a child, can get while also stressing condoms as the primary method of protection, this episode becomes an exemplar of how easily the topic can be discussed. Unfortunately, the same cannot be said of a more recent episode of the series.

Airing almost exactly one year later, on October 15, 2009, the episode "Right Here Right Now" introduces sisters, one of whom is in desperate need of the other's kidney. The hitch is that the donor sister is HIV-positive. This is the extent of the discussion of the issue. Viewers watch as the doctors proceed to debate if they should do the transplant neglecting to offer any information beyond the fact that she would be giving AIDS to her sister.

We never learn how the sister became positive, which could work to increase viewers' perceptions of their own vulnerabilities. In fact, the episode actually seems to move a few steps backward in challenging common perceptions by blatantly stating, "AIDS is no longer a death sentence. We have drugs now, it's no big deal" (*Private Practice S3 E3*). Moreover, not only does this episode miss the opportunity to affect viewer perceptions of how habits can affect health outcomes or increase perceptions of personal vulnerability or risk, but it inadvertently reinforces the idea that, thanks to modern medicine, HIV/AIDS is "no big deal."

Treichler (1999) observes that medical dramas on television typically are credited with serving a number of cultural functions. First is that they give disease a "human face." In the case of HIV/AIDS, this face remains that of homosexual men and prostitutes, which, in many ways, could be perpetuating ongoing stigma toward members of these populations as well as feeding the perception that most young viewers are not at risk. Medical dramas are also thought to portray the world of medicine and disease realistically, educating viewers on the issues presented. However, as discovered in this analysis, while some facts were presented about HIV, many misperceptions were also perpetuated, allowing for the miseducation of viewers. Finally, these dramas allow the television industry to entertain with a serious social edge, engaging the viewer imaginatively with contemporary social issues. This point is as true today as it was in the past; however, given that HIV and AIDS continue to be a social issue, it should be the role of these shows to normalize routine HIV testing as well as presenting factual information.

Crime/Legal Dramas

Although some of the medical dramas discussed above included legal aspects surrounding HIV, for the crime/legal procedural subgenre the focus is less on the repercussions of a doctor's choices and more on the use of HIV as a weapon or repercussion of poor choices. Multiple episodes of 17 shows,[6] were examined. For most, the HIV/AIDS narrative was contained within one or two episodes. However, for the HBO series *Oz* HIV played a unique central storyline to the entire series.

Providing a glass window to look through is about the only protection *Oz* provided the viewer. Between graphic situations, including prison rape, gang attacks, and complex topics of life and death *Oz* introduces the audience into a world not of munchkins and a lost teen girl, but of the gruesome world of one maximum security prison. The series takes place in Oswald State Correctional Facility, a fictional prison in upstate New York. Commonly referred to as the Emerald City,[7] the prison is an extremely controlled environment, with a unique assortment of prisoners from each racial and social group. The inclusion of the various groups is intended to provide conflict and tensions among these various factions; however, there is another story arc that plays a significant role in the series. The prison's own AIDS ward provides a number of narrative plotlines throughout the series. In some episodes the ward itself is used as punishment: when an inmate displays clear homophobia physically attacking another inmate. In another episode working in the AIDS ward is used as means of acquiring HIV-infected blood for the purpose of infecting another prisoner. Though not a primary thread to every episode, *Oz* provides the widest range of HIV/AIDS narratives, with nearly all focusing on the most horrific aspects of dying from the disease, framing HIV as a punishment (both in terms of having to work with those with it, as well as direct dialogue about AIDS being a punishment for misdeeds), and the use of HIV to harm other inmates (through either rape or injections). *Oz* however was not the first to explore the concern of people using HIV as a weapon.

The depiction of HIV and AIDS as a punishment served as a common theme throughout many of the shows regardless of genre. However, the specific use of HIV to punish others was unique to the crime/legal subgenre. For example, in 1998 *Law and Order* aired an episode titled "Carrier." In the episode Kenny Stark, a young HIV-positive man seeks to infect as many women as possible, "he bragged about infecting as many girls as he could, saying he would take us all down with him." Throughout the episode the topic of testing, treatment, and prevention are mentioned yet the larger concern centers upon the idea of whether knowingly giving someone an illness like HIV could/should be considered a criminal act. From the perspective of the prosecution, Stark is seeking out people to hurt and is knowingly infecting anyone who engages in unprotected sex. However, given that such a trial could start a witch hunt for anyone who passes HIV to another person, the local AIDS advocacy groups urged the lawyer in charge of the case not to push forward, "If you move forward with this case you're crucifying an entire community." Responding to the fact that Kenny was not gay, executive A.D.A. Jack McCoy (Sam Waterston) is confronted with the fact that "when people hear AIDS they think gay. The tabloids will use this case to attack anyone who is HIV positive. Which includes gays."

In 2010 *Law and Order: Special Victims Unit* revisited the topic of knowingly passing HIV to people in the episode "Quickie" (S11 E11). In the episode, a young man with an online alias of "Big Peter" employs multiple online hook-up applications to sleep with as many women as possible. Bragging about knowing his status and still not using condoms, he is brought into the precinct. Given that this episode took place years after the previously mentioned episode, the district attorney explains that charging "Big Peter" with attempted murder is not unprecedented and that "a court in Texas just put a man away for 45 years for infecting six women." In the end, both shows go to trial, and the men are prosecuted. Though the women's lives would remain forever altered, the shows end with a sense that justice was served.

Seeking justice for those impacted by HIV was also seen in two other shows: *The Equalizer* and *21 Jump Street.* Each approached the topic of HIV with a frame of protection. Airing in the late 80s both episodes focused on the protection of a young boy, or teen in the case of *21 Jump Street*, from outsiders presenting physical harm. Additionally, the protector in each episode was someone who needed to remain covert. For six-year-old Mickey

Robertson (played by Corey Carrier), protection is needed from the local men who continuously try to threaten him and his grandmother upon discovering he has HIV. In the *21 Jump Street* episode, "A Big Disease with a Little Name," Harley Poolish (played by Philip Tanzini) is given protection while attending his third high school since receiving his HIV diagnosis. In the beginning, it is made known both of these characters contracted the virus from blood transfusions; however, this is not where the similarities end, and it is also not entirely the truth for one of the young men.

In this emotionally tense and information-packed episode, *21 Jump Street* introduces the audience to a sarcastic and wild teen. On the surface, Harley shows little concern for life now that he knows he will die. Harley states, "Look pal, there is something you need to understand. A guy with a death sentence doesn't really worry about breaking any laws" (*21 Jump Street* S2 E13). After slowly gaining Harley's trust, undercover cop Hanson, Johnny Depp's character, discovers the painful truth that happens when you live with HIV. In one of the first emotional scenes Harley explains to Hanson, "You know I wasn't always such a horse's ass. But dead men don't make friends easily. Especially with kids who don't think they are ever going to die. I just wish they weren't so afraid to even touch me. Nobody touches me anymore, man. Not my dad; hardly even my mom. It's the worst part." This internal struggle, and feeling that he will never experience touch or love again Harley tells Hanson his plans to commit suicide: "You know how you beat AIDS? Don't let it kill you first. And when you are not happy anymore. You take yourself out." Fortunately, Harley did in fact have people who loved him and on the day of the planned event Hanson meets Harley and they embrace in a climatic hug of friendship and hope.

Across nearly all of the episodes analyzed within this subgenre, stigma, fear, and discrimination toward people living with HIV provided a central theme. Many characters portrayed with HIV or AIDS contract it from drugs or sex and most pass away from either the illness or another cause by the end of the episode. Those living with HIV are beaten up, ostracized, dropped from insurance companies, and fired from places of employment. For example, in the 2006 episode "Expectations" of *Without a Trace* (S4 E19), an HIV-positive pregnant woman faces judgment and discrimination from a lab technician while collecting a blood sample. "Oh, I don't judge. But God does. To be so selfish, and put an innocent child at risk." Comments about the judgment of God on behavior were one thing, but other shows took the role of "judge" to a new level. One of the worst examples of violent acts against people living with HIV was seen in a 1990 episode of *Law and Order* titled "Reaper's Helper" (S1 E3), when the antagonist targets and murders people living with HIV. His justification, he was "cleansing" the city of its "filth."

The depiction of people living with HIV as "filth" or being "dirty" was also observed in episodes of *Hill Street Blues* and *NYPD Blue*. Serving only as secondary, even tertiary storylines, the HIV-positive characters in each of the episodes were shown as homeless, sick, and literally filthy. Having past history, either as an informant or friend of the past, each of the men are "looked after" by a central character. Unfortunately for each, this friendship would not be enough, as they both pass away. In both cases, HIV serves only as a brief mention when explaining a character's backstory. Little information about how the virus is contracted is discussed, although it can be implied. For both men, life post–HIV status is melancholy and hopeless. In cases where HIV is simply mentioned, it begs the question, what is the purpose of mentioning it at all? The danger in these types of episodes is that all the viewer can observe is the stereotype of who contracts HIV and destruction that it causes.

More so than the other subgenres of dramatic narratives, crime and legal dramas require the audience to complete their own forms of deductive analysis in order to gain knowledge about HIV. For the majority of these narratives, few facts or medical information is presented in any of the shows examined. One episode, however, did present a variety of HIV medical information. In season 10 (2008) of *Law and Order: SVU* a great deal of attention was given to addressing the many myths and conspiracies surrounding HIV. The episode "Retro" begins with the investigation of an "abandoned" HIV-infected baby. As the episode progresses, the integrative team uncovers that the child's mother had left the child with her neighbors, who didn't know the child had HIV. When the child becomes ill, the neighbors recognize the symptoms and take the child to the fire station. Once the child's mother is discovered to be serving time in jail it becomes evident that she had not understood the importance of retroviral medication prior to birth and thus unknowingly passed the virus to her child. When the neighbors, who had taken the baby in, were asked why they didn't seek treatment for the child, they reply, "because the medicine is poison" (*Law and Order: SVU* S10 E5).

According to the president of Gambia, the small West African country the couple was originally from, HIV could be cured by rubbing a green paste on the positive person's chest, drinking a dose of bitter brew, and eating two bananas. Now living in the United States the couple sought the help of a local doctor who also believed that HIV could be cured through herbs, vitamins, even yogurt—but not from the poison the government was using to hurt people as part of a larger government conspiracy. As a result, the investigation identifies a number of patients, including a young teen boy, who have continued to go without treatment. Throughout the episode, multiple facts about HIV are presented including a video explaining how HIV impacts the body and information about treatment advances, resulting in a direct educational experience that attempts to dispel many conspiracies present today.

For the next six years the HIV narrative vanishes from criminal/legal genre. Offering a new take on the crime subgenre the 2014 smash hit *How to Get Away with Murder* reintroduces the topic of HIV. Knowing his partners colorful past, Oliver Hampton, played by Conrad Ricamora, engages in an open conversation about the need for testing with his partner Connor. Unlike the previous shows mentioned *How to Get Away with Murder* does not introduce HIV in the form of a client. Instead, it is woven into the story of one of the secondary characters. In the season one finale Oliver confronts Connor stating, "We need to get tested. You were a drug addict, and you cheated on me. And how many guys has your penis touched?" (S1 E15). With some convincing, "think about how great the sex will feel when we don't have to worry," the couple go together to get tested. Not only does this episode provide lengthy discussion of why testing is needed, but they also show the couple going together to do the testing.

The storyline presented provides both medially accurate information, "No. That is incorrect. Being 'on top' has the same risk of being on the bottom," but also given the judgment exuded from the medical provider the scene illustrates the continued stigma surrounding HIV. Thus, this scene highlights one of the barriers to testing: fear of judgment. The testing scene overall provided an accurate depiction of the risk questions, and the general uncomfortability one feels when getting tested. But as a means of helping to encourage people to get tested, the nurse's overall manner should have been far more encouraging or supportive.

For legal and crime shows the conflict presented in a show is limited by the case needing to be solved. With such a format, it is not surprising that the show's writers would be on a constant lookout for current events and topics to thread into the narrative. Thus, the manner through which HIV was seen in the narratives was also unsurprising. Yet, an inherent danger in framing HIV as the "evil" that must be resolved is that viewers will not want to identify with those characters. Instinctually, viewers will likely watch these narratives and see only the drug use, rape victims, and promiscuity. Thinking to themselves, "I am not that person and those things will not happen to someone like me." However, given that a viewer of this genre is likely seeking the thrill of solving the puzzle, it is possible that viewers wouldn't accept educational fodder from this format even when they do identify with a character.

Teen Dramas

Consistent with previous research (Gavin 2001; Treichler 1999), the teen drama subgenre was found to provide the most consistent amount of educational moments in terms of sexual health. Looking across the variety of teen dramas, many sexual health topics (including teen pregnancy, STIs, birth control, etc.) have been covered. However, only four shows (*Degrassi High*

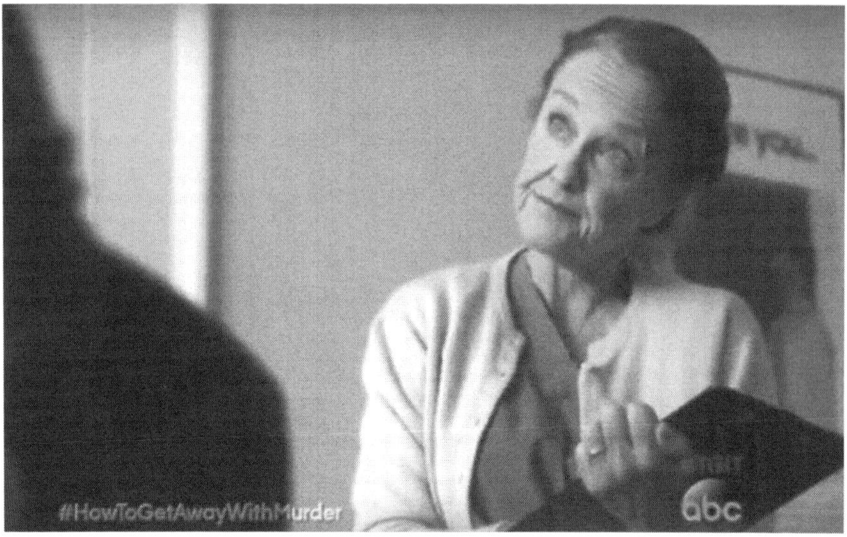

Figure 4.1. ***How to Get Away with Murder*, "The Night Lila Died; It's All My Fault Part 1" (2015). Source: ABC Studios**

[*DH*], *Beverly Hills, 90210*, *Dawson's Creek*, and *90210*)[8] specifically discussed HIV directly. These shows offered viewers examples of the dangers of risky behaviors, conversations about testing, as well as insight into the common fears and concerns anyone experiences while waiting for results. These shows also followed a consistent narrative structure in the ways HIV is brought into the show, the lessons presented, and even the ways the characters speak about their fears. For example, *Degrassi High* (*DH*), an early 90s Canadian-based show airing on PBS, hit audiences hard with an honest and direct discussion of HIV when 16-year-old Dwayne Myers, played by Darrin Brown, discovers he has contracted HIV from a summer fling.

The two-part storyline primarily focuses on the internal struggle of wondering if he has HIV, and what this will mean for his future. Throughout the show, facts about the need to use protection are presented from teachers, the medical provider conducting the test, as well as from Dwayne himself. However, while the show provides factual information about testing, the viewer also observes the negative connotations of HIV as a fellow student, upon discovering his secret, blackmails Dwayne. Dwayne also speaks directly of the idea of HIV as a punishment. "I didn't do anything wrong, I was just careless, and now I am going to suffer" (*Degrassi High*, S2 E2). As if following a teen drama template, each of the other episodes examined, including *Beverly Hills, 90210*, *Dawson's Creek*, and *90210*, each followed suit by having a sexual partner from the past return to deliver the episode shattering news that they were HIV-positive and a character the audience adored would need to be tested. Unlike *DH*, however, all of the other characters would test negative thus ending the HIV narrative.

Given continued challenges in providing comprehensive sex education to young adults within the United States, shows targeted at this population have a unique opportunity to imbed educational moments in the narrative. Messages should be short, focused, and careful not to come across as a lecture; however, anytime young people are shown discussing or engaging in sexual behaviors prevention of HIV and STIs should be included. Young people are rarely given the opportunity to see people talking about testing or protection. Thus, something as simple as showing a condom wrapper or including a conversation about testing, as seen in other subgenres, could have a profound effect on young viewers.

Daytime Dramas

Unlike the majority of serial dramas, viewers of soap operas are given opportunities to engage with the fictional worlds of their favorite soap opera on a daily basis. Given that soap operas often take on popular social issues it was no surprise when NBC's *Another World* introduced Dawn Rollo, played by Barbara Tyson. Dawn's story was the first AIDS-related storyline on a daytime soap opera in the United States airing in 1987. Dawn's character was short lived when she contracted HIV from a blood transfusion and died of AIDS in 1988.

A few years later, HIV returned to the soap opera screen when ABC's *General Hospital*, the longest running American soap opera currently in production, introduced two HIV-positive characters. Robin Scorpio, played by Kimberly McCullough, discovers she has contacted the virus from her boyfriend Stone Cates, played by Michael Sutton. The tragic relationship between Stone and Robin, and consequently HIV/AIDs, became such an important storyline that it even inspired one of the show's most famous events, the annual Nurses' Ball. This fictional gala continues to pay tribute to the characters while also raising awareness and funds for HIV and AIDS research. Although Stone dies of AIDS in the early 90s, Robin lived on until 2012, when a murderous stalker kept Robin from properly taking her meds, causing her drug regimen to fail. Ultimately, Robin's character, the first feature character to test HIV-positive within a show, exposed viewers to the HIV-positive life by openly discussing antiretrovirals,[9] safe sex, and prevention of mother-to-child transmission.

Although daytime dramas offer more frequent exposures to health narratives, viewership is often limited to people who are home during the day. For viewers who are not fans of soap operas, but still seek to immerse themselves into a world of conflict and drama, evening serial dramas airing weekly are the next best thing. Similar to soap operas, viewers are given featured characters watched on a weekly basis. However, unlike soap operas the conflict creating the drama is often limited to one or two episodes. Thus, most commonly the conflict is created by a secondary character, often a celebrity guest appearance. Similar to the made-for-TV movies and soap operas conflict plays a central role in the storyline. However, the type of conflict occurring will be based on the subgenre the show falls into.

Even More Drama

For viewers who seek to move past the somewhat predictable high school teen drama, yet are not interested in daytime dramas, a variety of other options simply labeled as American dramas provide the last, somewhat miscellaneous, grouping of shows containing HIV narratives. These dramas include thirtysomethings (*Melrose Place*, *Thirtysomething*, *Queer as Folk*, *Looking*), families (*Picket Fences*, *Life Goes On*, *Everwood*, *Brothers and Sisters*), politics and military (*Commander in Chief*, *JAG*), and an ex-cop turned late night radio show host (*The Midnight Caller*). Although each show might target a variety of audiences, the manner through which HIV is discussed in the show was found to be less varied.

For most of the shows, it's the same old story. A partner from the past reemerges with the news that they have contracted HIV. Luckily for the straight characters this test will be prove to be negative and the show will move along. However, for an unlucky few—the gay characters in *Picket Fences*, *Life Goes On*, *Brothers and Sisters*—the test will come back positive. While this storyline was common among the shows, a few episodes did choose an alternative path.

Take for instance in *The Midnight Caller*, airing in December of 1988 on Lifetime, Gary Cole, playing the character Jack Killian, receives a call from a girlfriend of his past. Discovering that she is pregnant, and has contracted HIV from a recent lover, she confides in Jack. "I feel like someone has just canceled the rest of my life" (*Midnight Caller* S1 E3), questioning herself saying, "How could I have been so stupid? I know the risks." Offering support Jack asks how "Mike," the man responsible, took the news. "That's the problem, I can't find him. . . . It's like he's disappeared." Finally, she asks for Jack's help, saying that "he has the right to know he might be sick."

At this point in the show, the concern and focus is on trying to help "Mike," however, this tone quickly shifts when Jack discovers that Mike has been dancing his way across the city spreading HIV to anyone, male and female, he can seduce into sleeping with him. Uncovering multiple victims of Mike's love, Jack engages in multiple conversations about the need to be tested, protecting others from the continued spread, and the need for support.

Unfortunately, not all are receptive; for instance, upon meeting Kelly, a woman Mike met at work, Jack is told she sees no need to get tested. "I don't think I want to know." Hearing this Jack replies, "In a way, I understand. But what about the damage you might be doing to others?" In turn Kelly ends the conversation stating, "Who ever thought about the damage they were doing to me?" Nearing the end of the episode Jack finally tracks Mike down and is able to confront him. During the course of the conversation Mike states:

> Do you have any idea what it's like to know you are going to stop breathing? Not someday, or when you get old, but this calendar year? Do you have any idea? Every meal, every sunrise, every woman, every man. I thirst to live life to the fullest. That's why I don't give up. . . . It's my life. It's all I have left. And I am going to make the best of the time I have left.

As the conversation continues, Jack tells Mike, "Ross sends you a message, he hopes God forgives you." As condescendingly as he has been throughout the scene Mike replies, "I wasn't very nice to Ross, bless his heart. But you see I believe that as long as hope remains you are safe from death. It's when you give into despair, when you allow the disease to beat us, that we finally die. And I don't want to die yet." As the screen fades to black, and the music fades, it's clear nothing Jack can say will stop this man from continuing his selfish desires, at least nothing he can say to Mike directly. Jack chooses to use the power of the airwaves and calls Mike out by name, description, and HIV status to all who are listening.

Ultimately, Jack's on-air discussion and nearly all of the dramatic shows open the line for important discussions about the fear and misperceptions people had about anyone with HIV and AIDS. Throughout many of the shows, meaningful conversations occurred between friends, family, and loved ones. Conventions modeling support, acceptance no matter what, as well as facts about HIV. For example, one of the best conversations about the fear and need for testing occurred during an episode of *Brothers and Sisters*.

From 2006 to 2011, viewers became part of the family as they watched ABC's weekly drama *Brothers and Sisters*. Similar to many other dramas the show tackles a number of social issues and topics as the affluent, and often political, Walker family attempts to move forward after the family patriarch's death. Inclusive of sexual orientation the show includes three gay primary characters, including Saul, played by Ron Rifkin, the brother of the now matriarch, Nora.

Discovering a past partner from over twenty years on Facebook, Saul does the math realizing their paths had crossed at a time when HIV could have been contracted. Sharing the concern with his nephew Kevin and his husband Scotty, Saul opens a conversation about testing for STIs and HIV. Not only is the conversation about testing one of the few to occur in dramatic shows; it also quickly and simply made the idea of getting tested normal. Saul casually asks if his nephews got tested; quickly and without any hesitation, Kevin shakes his head yes while Scotty replies, "For HIV, of course. It's like habit not unlike spring cleaning" (*Brothers and Sisters* S4 E24). This comparison of testing as an annual habit not only echoes the suggestions of the CDC and other public health officials, but it also offers viewers the opportunity to see testing as a normalized activity, and not something to be scared about. As seen as the conversation continued, Saul, like most, is still concerned about the test. He mentions to his nephews that he is sure if he had something he would know by now. "I am like 100 years old, I would know by now." Thus, offering yet another common misperception viewers may have. Feeling concerned the couple later brings up the testing conversation with Saul again, finally convincing him to seek out testing the next time he is at the doctor.

When the conversation with the medical provider occurs, viewers are provided one of the most supportive and nonjudgmental conversations aired. The scene begins with Saul again making note of his age and how it must be surprising to see someone like him seeking testing. Without missing a beat, the nurse smiles and says, "I wish we did. The over-50 age-set is our fastest rising risk group." Still questioning the likelihood of being asymptomatic Saul finally directly asks the nurse if someone can have HIV and not know, even decades later. Thus, for a second time the audience is given information about the dangers of thinking you would "know" you had the virus.

The nurse in the scene not only provided basic facts but more importantly her manner throughout the discussion remained calm and compassionate. Typical for anyone getting tested the following "hours" for Saul were filled with visible uncertainty. Unfortunately for Saul, the call the following day would only confirm his greatest fears. Even more unfortunate is that viewers would only be able to observe the healthy portrayals and positive experiences including reconnecting with his previous partner, falling in love, and deciding to get married in the remaining episodes as the show came to an emotional close.

HIV CONFLICT ACROSS GENRES

One of the pinnacle components of drama, regardless of the subgenre, is the inclusion of conflict. Be it internal (conflict within one's self), external (conflict occurring between two or more people), or environmental conflict, all dramas rely on some form as a primary means of moving a story along and keeping an audience hooked. It is said that without conflict there would be no story. This is especially true within the dramatic narratives, which is why including a plotline of HIV within a show should not be surprising. As with almost any major medical concern the most common type of conflict is the internal struggle of "do I have it?" Subsequently, then the question becomes "what would this mean for my life?" However, given the withstanding stigma surrounding HIV and AIDS additional questions of "who do I trust," "how do I tell my family and friends," as well as "will anyone ever love me again" become increasingly important.

Internal Conflict

Looking across the shows analyzed within this genre the internal conflict of "do I have it" was resoundingly the most common. Be it sparked from an ex-partner returning from the past, a mysterious illness, or engagement with someone outside of a relationship, the request, or need, to obtain an HIV test instantly ignites deep-seated fears. This form of conflict, however, is a ubiquitous experience. Most people when faced with the possibility of testing positive for an illness would be consumed with worry. What makes the experience of testing for HIV a driver for conflict is the sequential struggles, for instance, the question "will this be my punishment for past behaviors?"

Given the nature of how HIV is transmitted, it is not surprising that numerous characters are shown battling internal demons and questioning personal choices. Regardless of age, gender, even sexual orientation characters can be heard not only questioning but also judging their own actions. For most characters this line of judgement occurs after sexual activity has taken place with someone outside of a relationship. In the earlier example, Dr. Caldwel (*St. Elsewhere* S4 E15) states, "I love women, Jack. That's why I am in this trouble now. I was always attracted to nice girls. But when I couldn't find them, I would lock my wallet and watch in the glove compartment and head into the combat zone." For Dr. Caldwel this combat zone included a prostitute, with an additional implied intravenous drug habit. However, even when sexual activity occurs with a partner, some characters, such as Kelly in *Midnight Caller* (S1 E3), are heard questioning themselves. "I knew the risks, how could I be so stupid?" Sex, however, was not the only "stupid" activity characters judged themselves for. In a 1993 episode of *NYPD Blue* Ferdinand Holley, played by Giancarlo Esposito, shares that he too "deserved what he got" given his past deeds saying, "It's not like I don't deserve this. You know all the shooting up I done" (*NYPD Blue*, S2 E7). Multiple characters across shows, decades, and subgenres echoed the feeling of HIV or AIDS being a punishment they deserved. This statement also mirrors the ways in which HIV had been portrayed in the news. News anchors, doctors, and politicians alike were quoted making comments about who was contracting the virus while passing judgement on the manner through which transmission had occurred.

Fear of possible stigma surrounding HIV, each of the characters portrayed with HIV were shown facing a multitude of internal struggles as they attempted to cope with living with the virus. For some, the struggle surrounded the fear of coworkers finding out their status. In the 2005 episode of *Commander in Chief* the concern about HIV became a political and public relations matter. Vince Taylor (Anthony Azizi) plays an aid to the President of the United States and when word surfaces that he has been living with HIV for over ten years he is faced with the fear that the opposition will use his status as a political tool. "You are not an average citizen. You are the special aid to the president. You're gay, you're infected, and you are news" (*Commander in Chief* S1 E7) a member of the opposing side warns. As a result, Taylor struggles with the decision of risking embarrassing the administration or resigning. In a similar manner both Dr. Caldwel (*St. Elsewhere*) and Dr. Boulet (*ER*) are challenged with the internal struggle of how living with the virus could impact their careers. However, for these characters the repercussions of living with the virus are not just about public relations or credibility, but more so the risk of being around patients. Occurring in the mid-1980s, and a time where little was known about the risks of transmission, Dr. Caldwel is forced to resign from his post at the hospital. Dr. Boulet on the other hand is able to remain working; however, she soon begins experiencing one of the most important internal conflicts, who can I trust in disclosing my status to?

The internal struggle of accepting that you are in fact living with any chronic illness is challenging enough, but for those with HIV it is more than simply a matter of managing the illness by taking medication and seeing a doctor annually. Those living with the virus are faced with the repeated questions of who do I have to disclose to; and more importantly, who can trust? The majority of shows only include one episode focused on HIV, with the dominant conflict being created by fear of testing. Thus, it is not surprising that far fewer episodes allowed viewers to witness the undertaking related to self-disclosure. As mentioned above Dr. Boulet (*ER*) was able to remain at the hospital where she worked. In part this was due to the fact that she had shared her status with a friend who actively helped to keep the status quiet. However, it was not long before others in the hospital discovered the secret and larger questions regarding her fit at the hospital were called. Yet beyond the workplace, the primary area for disclosure is within a relationship.

Telling a previous partner about one's status was by far the most common theme found within the area of disclosure. What is rarely seen, however, is the internal struggle those characters go through prior to doing so. Far less common was the inclusion of someone with HIV talking to a new potential partner about their status. The first ever show to include a continued HIV-positive character,[10] and one of the earliest depictions of a status disclosure to a potential partner, was the show *Life Goes On.* Jesse (Chad Lowe) begins as a platonic friend of Becca Thacher, played by Kellie Martin. Near the end of the series the relationship intensifies, resulting in Jesse's disclosure of his HIV. Pulling on the viewers heart strings multiple scenes explicitly display the fear and worry related to telling someone you care about you have a life-threatening illness. Since this airing, few shows have included a repeated character living with the virus and even fewer include the internal conflict how to tell a potential partner about their status. In fact, only two shows (*Queer as Folk*, *Looking*) stood out as including such conversations. In both cases the audience themselves (more often members of the LGBTQ community) would likely already be accustomed to these conversations.

External Conflict

With quick and harsh judgment being passed on people due to the means of transmission, it stands to reason that the second most common form of conflict focused on external conflict. From previous partners returning with a warning, medical providers giving results, and people discovering the status of those around them, bringing in an HIV narrative opens multiple possibilities for heated and tense conversations.

The most obvious external conflict one might expect might be a previous partner disclosing their status (suggesting a test, this was not found to be the case) or the discovery of one's status. In the few instances where this scenario is shown, the tensions are high in the scene and the tone of the moment is always tense, but characters were rarely shown getting into a conflict. In almost every case the conversation occurs and the internal conflict begins. The only occurrence of external conflict igniting when a character discovers they have HIV was found in the episode "It's a Family Thing" of the show *Private Practice* (S1 E2). Having known and lied to their son about his "illness" his entire life, Dr. Cooper is forced to push the parents to tell their son the truth when it is mentioned to the doctor that the teen is planning to have sex with his girlfriend on prom night. In this situation the conflict occurs not only with the parents about the need to be open and honest with their child, but also between the teenager and Dr. Cooper. Upon discovering the truth Dean erupts at Dr. Cooper screaming, "You knew. And all this time you didn't tell me. I thought you were my friend." Feeling betrayed by his parents and doctor, Dean's internal conflict becomes even more complicated by the fact that by the time he was finally told, he and his girlfriend had already had sex. The external conflict is left implied when Dean, the girlfriend, and the girlfriend's parents return to the clinic the following day stating, "What you said about answering questions. We have a lot." The look of concern and anger specifically on the father's face makes it clear there had been a great deal of heated conversation prior to getting to the clinic.

A parent's primary job is always to protect their child from harm. Knowing the stigma surrounding HIV, Dean's parents explicitly stated that their choice of not disclosing his status drew from fear of what would happen to him, "Do you have any idea what it is like for HIV kids? A kid in Chicago got shot. And another kid, they tied him to a car bumper." Look across the episodes of teens dealing with an HIV status and it is clear that Dean's parents might have been correct. Frequently characters, especially young characters, living with the virus are shown struggling with bullying, discrimination, verbal threats, and physical violence.

Bullying in some cases, for instance, for the character in *21 Jump Street*, was so bad he was forced to leave multiple schools, create a more palatable story to explain his infection, and hire an undercover cop as protection. Harvey's character, however, was not alone. In the 1987 show *The Equalizer* it was a six-year-old boy who required protection. Contracting AIDS from his mother, Mickey Robertson, played by Corey Carrier, faces extreme levels of bullying (including his home being broken into and belongings destroyed). After having moved to yet another new neighborhood the young boy's diagnosis is discovered by the locals and soon it is clear for his own protection he and his grandmother, and caregiver, will be forced to move; that is, until the show's hero gets involved. For Dywane Myers (Darrin Brown), in a 1989 episode of *Degrassi High*, the discovery of his HIV status not only results in being blackmailed by a fellow student, but also a bloodied face as he is attacked in the high school bathroom.

Environmental Conflict

Though multiple characters experienced physical harm to themselves and their property, the stigma surrounding HIV and AIDS was most commonly observed in the form of discrimination. Echoing the events taking place off screen, characters were shown battling the environments in which they lived. Although environmental conflict is more often thought of in terms of natural disasters, it also manifests as political, social, economic, ethnic, religious, or territorial conflicts. In other words, conflicts occurring due to a lack of resources or difference in national interests.

Losing jobs, places to live, and refusal of treatment by medical and police personnel characters in multiple shows illuminated the alarming non-medial aspects of living with HIV and AIDS. In the episode "The Venus Butterfly" of *LA Law* a juror is asked how they feel about being in a room with someone who is HIV-positive, to which she states, "The truth is, I would rather not be in room every day with a guy that's got it" (S1 E10). Thankfully, given that the client was indeed HIV-positive, that juror was removed from trial. However, the remainder of the episode continued to highlight the blatant discrimination people living with the virus face every day. Throughout the episode the question became, does a terminal patient have the right to take their own life if they know they will die soon anyway? The client on trial aided in the death of his partner after facing multiple medial and insurance barriers. Airing in the decade ripe with fear and misunderstanding, comments such as “AIDS is a biblical punishment, plagued to the gay community” were not surprising, nor was the jury’s guilty of first degree murder verdict.

DECADES OF DRAMA: LOOKING AT HIV THEMES ACROSS TIME

It’s not at all surprising that so many shows would elect to include narratives of HIV within the drama genre. A point made clear by the fact that in none of the shows did the topic of HIV ever feel forced or out of place. Yet while the many of the plotlines for bringing HIV into the show have seen little evolution, the same cannot be said of the tone of the episodes. In the beginning of the epidemic the tone across all genres and platforms was one of fear. As discussed in chapter three, news programs and headlines were riddled with words such as “death,” “cancer,” and “plague.” Following suit, the dramas themselves also focused on the ultimate death sentence that was HIV. Characters in the 80s and early 90s were almost always shown, or implied, dying by the end of the episode. As medical advances and understanding increased, characters were consequently shown living longer. Depicting characters living with the virus not only offered opportunities to provide more awareness and education but has also altered the mood of the episodes.

Holding on to the seriousness of HIV, the need to get tested, and the idea that anyone regardless of sexual orientation could be at risk, shows throughout the years have continued to provide a tense and emotional experience for the viewers. Regrettably, the intensity and urgency once felt in the early 80s and 90s has since lessened as time has gone on. With new drug cocktails and prevention advancements people are able to live long lives with the virus. Thus, modern narratives no longer need to focus on the almost certain death. Instead, shows now focus on the challenges of living with a spreadable and still stigmatized chronic illness. For instance, concerns from friends and family who would not understand, the myriad of health considerations, and legal troubles have become the common topics aligned with HIV.

Even though the most recent episodes highlight the anxiety that naturally comes with testing for HIV, little is shown in terms of the stigma still felt by many who actually live with the illness. In the rare instance that an HIV-positive character is given multiple episodes, HIV only becomes a topic of conversation when sex, blood, or a legal concern is apparent. Little is ever mentioned about the other realities people living with HIV face including mental health, having to reshape an identity, travel restrictions, or the challenging decisions about disclosure to potential partners and places of work. In fact, only two shows, *ER* and *Commander in Chief*, spent any time highlighting the workplace disclosure discussions. Additionally, *ER* was the only show to directly call attention to the financial cost of living with HIV. Other shows implied the burden of cost by showing HIV characters as homeless or having to go to free clinics for care, but for even slightly affluent characters, cost is never addressed.

What is provided in nearly every HIV narrative, across each decade, is some form of fact about HIV. The writers overall have done an effective job weaving in facts about risk, likelihood of passing the virus from mother to child, and overall transmission. Shows provided important lessons that it's not only gay populations that need to be concerned, but that everyone is at risk. Similarly, the shows offer a consistent narrative that HIV impacts not only those with the illness but also the people who know them. What has become disappointing in recent times is both the lack of conversation and the return to an almost exclusive portrayal of HIV as a gay disease.

Over forty shows were examined for this chapter of which eight aired after 2000. In the last four years, only two shows, *How to Get Away with Murder* and HBO's *Looking*, have taken on the topic of HIV. As a result, it has become far more difficult for people to hear facts about HIV, see people they could connect to getting tested, and more importantly observe the conversations between partners and support systems about risks.

NOTES

1. Medical dramas examined included *St. Elsewhere* (1986), *Chicago Hope* (1995), *ER* (1999), *Nip/Tuck* (2005), *House, MD* (2005), *Grey's Anatomy* (2008 and 2010), *Private Practice* (2008 and 2009).
2. For this episode AIDS was used throughout the show. For each show I will use the nomenclature used by the show. Discussion of the use of HIV vs. AIDS will be discussed in chapter seven.
3. Reuben continues to be an HIV advocate and speaker for groups such as the Minnesota AIDS Project forum in Minneapolis and Elizabeth Glaser Pediatric AIDS Foundation. She has also participated in World AIDS Day and she's a board member for the U.S. Sexuality Information and Education Council.
4. This form of treatment at one time was an accurate description of Heimlich's actual theories.
5. Expert from a four-page letter to the late Laurence Tisch, then CEO of CBS by Dr. Paul Bronston, an ER doctor and chair of a medical ethics board who has been among Heimlich's most outspoken critics. http://www.hollywoodreporter.com/news/chicago-hope-dealt-heimlich-malariotherapy-725010.
6. Crime/legal shows analyzed included *L.A. Law* (1986, 1991), *The Closer*, *The Equalizer* (1987), *21 Jump Street* (1988), *NYPD Blue*, *New York Undercover* (1996), *OZ*, *Law and Order* (1990), *Law and Order: SVU*, *New York Undercover*, *Without a Trace*, *Boston Legal*, *Commander in Chief*, *CSI: NY*, *Hill Street Blues*, *Murder One*, and *JAG*.
7. A setting from *The Wonderful Wizard of Oz* (1900).

8. *90210* was a 2008 spin-off of the original *Beverly Hills, 90210*. While none of the characters from the original show appeared in the new version, many of the central plotlines were similar.

9. The drugs used to treat HIV are called *antiretroviral* drugs. There are several different types and they work in different ways. http://www.who.int/hiv/topics/treatment/en/.

10. A total of six episodes were included during the last season of the show. Issues of disclosure, stigma, "gay" bashing, and ultimately the death of Jesse's character.

Chapter Five

HIV as a Punchline

Comedic Narratives on Stage and Screen

Narratives focusing on HIV and AIDS are likely to feel normal within a medical or legal/procedural drama. It's logical to talk about the symptoms and consequences of risky behaviors in shows with a more serious tone. But, can HIV be funny? Or as proposed by the writers of *South Park* have we reached the time when "AIDS is finally funny"? For a number of comedians, it would appear we have in fact reached that moment. The larger question is, at what cost? Does making HIV the punchline of a joke diminish the severity people attribute to the illness? Can incorporating HIV into a situational comedy provide emotional connection and facts about HIV? After examining three areas of the comedic genre: situational comedy, satire, and stand up, it seems that while HIV might at first come off as the punchline, in numerous instances discussions of HIV within a comedic genre have served as an important vehicle for prevention messaging. Such messages are especially present when writers work in collaboration with outside organizations. In such cases, shows are found to significantly contribute to dispel common misperceptions while raising HIV awareness. Following a similar format of the previous chapter the following begins a brief overview of the narrative elements found within the comedic genre.

STRUCTURES WITHIN THE COMEDY GENRE

Primarily running for 30 minutes each week the comedy genre provides viewers an escape into a world where no matter the situation a laugh can be offered. From witty dialogue, humorous situations, and even the use of physical comedy this genre has entertained audiences beginning in the 1950s with shows such as *I Love Lucy* and *The Honeymooners*. The most popular comedic formats on television being situational comedies (sitcoms), which include a variety of characters, with one or two taking the lead. Often mirroring or challenging social norms, what makes these shows funny are the topics and situations we see in everyday life. Although each real-life situation is likely played out in the most extreme way possible.

Gender, and sexually based, stereotypes are also a prominent framework within sitcoms. For example, a single man will be depicted as the forever bachelor, seeking sex, money, and power. While women are commonly shown obsessed with finding her perfect match, or if she is career focused then will have no time for romance. Stereotypes surrounding gay couples are also common with a focus on design- or entertainment-related careers and always having a flare for the dramatic.

Similar to the dramas evaluated in chapter four situational comedies also tend to rely on the "problem of the week" plot structure. This structure begins with everything seeming fine for the characters until some dilemma appears. Commonly, the "drama" or conflict for the shows revolves around dating/relationship or family life. For the single characters the dramas focus on needing dates, and dates going horribly wrong. For the couples, conflict centers on misunderstandings: men being "men," women "over reacting," or awkwardness in the bedroom. Thus, with so much comedy focusing on the romantic relationships of characters it's no surprise to see STIs and HIV interwoven into the story.

The most iconic example of HIV in the comedic genre came from sassy and voracious women of the 80s in *Designing Women*. After the writer, director, and producer of *Designing Women* Linda Bloodworth-Thomason's own mother had contracted AIDS from a blood transfusion, she witnessed first-hand the "incredible prejudice and prevailing ignorance inflicted not just on her, but all the homosexual men who shared her hospital floor."[1] Sitting at her mother's bedside she remarks in an interview with GLADD, "One day I overheard a woman in the hall say, "If you ask me, this disease has one thing going for it. It's killing all the right people." "Furious she took pen to paper and began writing what quickly became the Emmy-nominated episode "Killing all the Right People" (*Designing Women* S2 E4).

In the episode the infamous women of Sugerbaker's Design, led by owner and found Julia Sugarbaker (Dixie Carter), her sister Suzanne Sugarbaker (Delta Burke), as well as friends and colleagues Mary Jo Shively (Annie Potts) and Charlene Frazier Stillfield (Jean Smart) are reunited with a friend of the family, Kendall (Tony Goldwyn). Visiting with a plan of more than reconnecting, Kendall asked the women to design his funeral. Kendall states, "I am dying, and I like your taste." Shocked, Charlene replies, "What do you mean you're dying, you are just a kid." Kendall: "I have AIDS."

Throughout the scene Kendall explains that he is gay, but quickly reminds the women (and the viewers) that anyone can be at risk. Kendall describes that during his more recent trip to the hospital he had a 65-year-old grandfather who got it from a blood transfusion on one side of him and on the other side and 18-year-old girl who got it from her boyfriend who got it from a girl he used to date. Seeing that this illness was killing many people who might be abandoned by family, or will simply not have support, he asks the designers to help create a funeral space that will be available for anyone to use. Over the course of the conversation a variety of facts and myths about risk and treatment are discussed directly. Kendall states he is on medication, but the reality is there is still so much research to be done, and his T-cells are getting lower.

Meanwhile during a PTA meeting at Mary Jo's daughter's school, a secondary plotline is revealed. During the meeting, the teachers and parents debate about how sexual education should be handled and if it is appropriate for teens to be given condoms. With both narratives focused on sexual health over 85 percent of the dialogue confronts sex in some manner. While the factual aspects are vital to raising awareness about STIs and HIV, it is the show's discussion about ignorance and stigma that made the show a standout above all other shows, even decades later.

Back at the design firm, a client asks Julia if Kendall is "the boy you are designing the funeral for?" When confirmed, Emma Jean, the client played by Camilla Carr, states, "Now I don't like to hurt anyone's feelings but if these boys hadn't been doing what they were doing they wouldn't be getting what's coming to 'em now," igniting a heated and powerful moment for the show.

Mary Jo: Emma Jean, gays aren't the only ones gettin it.

Emma Jean: No, but they are the ones who started it.

Kendall: Actually no one knows how it got started. Gays are just the first group it showed up in.

Emma Jean: And for a good reason. You reap what you sow, and you boys brought this on yourselves. As far as I'm concerned this disease has one thing going for it. It's killing all the right people.

Furious Julia immediately asks another character to move their car because Emma Jean needed to leave. Insulted Emma Jean fires back a look of confusion. In true Sugerbaker fashion, Julia doesn't miss a beat explaining, "The one thing worse than all these people who never had morals before AIDS, is you holier than thou types who think you are exempt from getting it." Now visibly shaking with anger Emma Jean continues, "Well for your information

I am exempt. I've never lived like those people (pointing at Kendall) and I don't care what you say, Julia Sugerbaker, I believe this is God's punishment for what they've done." With the majority of people dying of AIDS being gay or drug users many people raised the question of this being the punishment you got for making poor choices. Thus, the show echoes the ongoing narrative of the 80s with the comment "God's punishment," and ignites a continued theme found across shows and decades especially within the comedic genre. Getting the final word Julia jumps in again, "Emma Jean get serious, who do you think you are talking to? I have known you for 27 years and all I can say is, if God was giving out sexually transmitted diseases to people as a punishment for sinning, then you would be at the free clinic all the time. (Emma Jean gasps and looks horrified.) And so would the rest of us." It is this exchange and the lines within it that sparked a great deal of conversation about how a show, especially one known for comedy, could address the serious topic of AIDS. In the remaining minutes of the episode Mary Jo finds her voice and speaks up at the PTA meeting about the need for teens to have access to sexual health education and condoms: "it's not just about preventing babies, it's about saving lives." In many ways the narrative presented in the show offered a direct call to action for viewers to wake up and understand that more was needed to prevent the continued rise of HIV, that anyone was at risk, and that AIDS was not a punishment. Though it may not be clear how many viewers were inspired to act, it is clear the episode did influence the writers of other shows with strong female characters to also speak up about prevention, testing, and stigma.

FEMALE FRIENDS AND CONVERSATIONS ABOUT HIV

With a title like *Sex and the City* it should not be surprising at all to find the topic of HIV. Especially when the show includes a character like Samantha, whose world revolves around casual sex. During season three of the show two episodes brought attention to the topic of testing for HIV and STIs. Directly taking on the topic of HIV a potential partner refuses to have sex with Samantha (Kim Cattrall), until she gets tested for HIV. In the episode, "Running with Scissors" (S3 E11), Samantha turns to her friends for advice asking bluntly, and without any warning, "Have you all had an AIDS test?" Shocked with eyes wide the friends look up from their meals and immediately look Samantha's way, "Good morning (almost choking), where did that come from?" one friend remarks; indicating the unexpectedness of the topic. Samantha begins to explain her predicament. Given Samantha's sexual escapades another friend calls into question the idea that it couldn't be possible that she, of all of them, had not been tested previously, "Wait a minute *you* have never had an HIV test?" Defensively, Samantha responds that she has not and asks the friends again if they have; to which two of the three explain they have at least a few times, the third refusing to engage in the conversation displaying her overall discomfort with the discussion. Again, Samantha is asked how it is possible that she of all of them has not been tested. As with many shows, as discussed later in chapter seven, often the character with a more colorful sexual history is used as the vehicle for discussing sexual health. However, in contrast to other shows Samantha is shown being the most fearful of obtaining the test; stating that her justification for not testing is her fear of finding out she has it. Quickly, and confidently, the friends reassure her that she will not "have it." Pushing back Samantha states "Sometimes it takes me a long time to recover from a cold." Thus, signifying some knowledge of how HIV impacts the body. Yet again the friends offer reassurances that Samantha will be "just fine" and encourage her to "Just go and get it over with. The test is nothing. The worst part is waiting for the results." In this moment the friends simply brush over Samantha's actual risk of HIV by reinforcing that she would be "fine" and couldn't have it. However, given her sexual history within the show they miss an important opportunity to discuss prevention methods. Comments such as "no big deal" and the immediate confirmation "you don't have it," regardless of past behaviors, minimize the severity of contracting a sexually transmitted illness.

Although airing on HBO, thus having a greater ability to openly discuss controversial topics such as the use of condoms, it is possible the writers felt the more palatable discussion would be on the anxiety of the test itself. As one friend, Carrie (Sarah Jessica Parker), explains the worst part of the test is the waiting. To this, Miranda (Cynthia Nixon) describes this experience, "Really! And then they come out with the results and motion to certain people and take them into the little room. And you know the news ain't good. I just sat there the entire time praying "please don't take me to the little room." Beyond this mention of the little room no additional information is offered about the test or Samantha's risk for testing positive. Thankfully, however, the show does include one of only five examples of a character going through the process of getting tested.

Throughout the testing process Samantha offers both insight to the types of questions typically asked about risk, but she also demonstrates the common fear and shame many feel when asked to evaluate previous sexual behaviors. Direct questions about the number of partners, types of activities engaged in, and the percentage of time using protection generates a few moments of laughter for the audience as Samantha's answers remain candid and light. Once such example is her response to the question, "Do you swallow?" during oral sex, to which she replies, "Only when surprised." Another moment of comedic relief is used in relation to the number of partners she has had. When the provider asks about the number of partners she looks up, and pauses, while her fingers demonstrate that she may be counting; making this point explicit she looks over seeing the provider's concerned look and states, "Oh . . . um. . . . I'm counting. Do you mean this year?"

This conversation provides the viewer a medically accurate dialogue while also addressing the very real discomfort of talking with a medical provider about sexual behavior. At the start, the audience observes the often-confident Samantha at a loss for words, yet as the questions continue she sees that there is little to no judgment coming from the medical provider. She assumes she will be judged, and even punished for her sexual history, however, by the end of the episode she is given a clean bill of health, and shown receiving her "prize" as she hooks up with the gentleman from the start of the episode.

Though, not directly focused on HIV an additional episode of *Sex and the City* should be discussed. Offering a strong focus on STIs, in "Are We Sluts?" (S3 E6), Miranda discovers during a routine doctor's checkup, that she has chlamydia. Although Miranda is sexually active throughout the show she casually states to her friend that this was her first test. As she continues, Miranda makes note of her feeling of being judged by the nurse when she is told to contact all of the people she might have given chlamydia to. The viewer is not privy to the actual conversation; however, perceived judgment from a provider was found to be a common theme across shows when testing or discussions about STIs and HIV were discussed.

Beginning the self-disclosure of her situation, Miranda bluntly states, "I can't tonight, I have chlamydia" just as her partner begins to initiate sexual activity. Confused, her partner responds, "I don't even know what that is, but it sounds like a problem." In attempts to ease his concern Miranda quickly dismisses the severity of contracting an STI explaining, "It's not a big deal. It's just a sexually transmitted disease. I might have given it to you, or you might have given it to me. Either way you need to get tested." Although she ends the remark with he should get tested, the comment "it's not a big deal" only encourages a mentality that STIs are not really something to worry about, and therefore why would the audience need to be concerned. The situation with Miranda is in some ways sobering, as the viewer observes that adults can be just as ignorant about their sexual health as most teenagers. At the same time, by highlighting the fear, discomfort, and shame the show could also motivate viewers not to get tested.

Both episodes, "Are We Sluts?" and "Running with Scissors," provide an informative narrative without ever coming across as an after school special. Given that Samantha, like all other female characters shown getting tested, is spared the lifelong consequences of HIV, and Miranda is shown with a curable illness, it becomes easy to balance the comedy and seriousness of STIs. Expectedly, both episodes present healthy and supportive peer conversations. Even when discussing testing over breakfast the women are shown offering emotional support and encouragement for getting the testing done.

Unfortunately, only one of the episodes takes advantage of the opportunities to model effective conversations with the partner about testing. Bringing Samantha back to his home within the span of five minutes, television time, Tom almost immediately asks, "So Samantha when was your last AIDS test?" Having never been tested he leans back and responsibly explains that while he really wants to proceed with the night's intended activities, he simply can't until he knows it is safe. Tom's directness and ability to stand firm that he wants to be safe can provide male viewers especially a model to follow. Female viewers are also able to see that getting tested is just as important.

For Miranda the conversations about the need to get tested take on a far more negative approach. The viewer is able to almost feel the level of embarrassment she experiences as she begins calling her past partners. Although statements such as "Sorry," "I know this is awkward," and "And congratulations! I guess now that you're married, you don't have to worry about stuff like this" do provide humor, they also exacerbate the awkwardness and ineffective methods of talking to a past partner about their risk. Additionally, both episodes miss vital opportunities for the medical providers to engage in discussion about prevention or routine testing.

A few years later, and on the other side of the country, another show featuring four girlfriends again took on the topic of HIV. Besides being demographically different in the character makeup, all four women being African American, the writers of the show *Girlfriends* also worked closely with the Henry J. Kaiser Family Foundation taking part in the yearlong campaign (KNOW HIV/AIDS) sponsored by UPN's parent company Viacom. Taking on the greatest risk, by not only including HIV into one episode but a total of four, *Girlfriends* provides effective messages about four different aspects of HIV.

Setting the stage for the longer focus, the first, and shortest, mention of HIV occurred in the episode "Take This Poem and Call Me in the Morning" (S3 E12). In the scene Savad (Saul Williams) performs what at first sounds like a deep in meaning, yet very sexual, poem. After the performance he tells one of the four primary characters, Lynn (Persia White), that it is not about sex at all, "It is about how AIDS is running rampant in Africa." Having heard Lynn is doing a documentary on Sex in LA, Savad challenges her to dig deeper and make an impact. "Girl, what I mean is how is it going to better us as people? Without purpose, it's just porn. OK, here is your topic, you're dying, Black women like you are dying. HIV is your killer. Document that." Without going into any statistics or directly offering any educational message, Savad is still able to draw attention to the very real reality that HIV is in fact the third leading cause of death for women of color.

Taking on the challenge Lynn does change her documentary's focus and begins to raise awareness and give voice to the one in three black women who will become HIV positive. One of whom she knows personally. Reesie (Kimberly Elise), a college friend, reconnects with the friends and discloses that her own husband gave her AIDS. In one scene the girls begin to ask Reesie about how it happened. Reesie explains that she contracted the virus from her husband who had sex with another man behind her back. When one of the friends questions the sexual orientation of her husband Reesie explains a common perception of men on the "down low" stating, "You see if he had put a condom in his pocket, that would have meant he would be admitting to himself that he was going out to have sex with men. That would make him gay. Which according to him he is not" (S3 E19). Of all of the mediated narratives examined thus far Reesie's story was the only one which addressed contracting HIV from a heterosexual partner who had engaged in same sex risky behavior. Reesie's storyline not only draws attention to the very real, and more common than what is portrayed on television, manner through which women contract HIV, but she also provides a powerful voice of how life altering living with HIV can be. Agreeing to be interviewed for Lynn's documentary she speaks directly to the camera with tears already welling up in her eyes,

> Being diagnosed with AIDS enhanced my perspective of living. A lot of people are ALIVE, but are not living. They're excited they are just here. Living is taking one tiny moment and making it turn into an eternity so you never lose it. It means putting a value on every breath you take so you might take another one. And I didn't view it that way . . . before I was diagnosed. (Sighs) Being told that I have AIDS had to be (stops) no it was the most terrifying moment in my life. It's not a moment that I asked for and I am not happy and I am not supposed to be but I have to deal with it. (Begins to really cry) And at times it's not the easiest thing to do.

Over the course of the four episodes the ladies of *Girlfriends* did far more than simply mention the topic of HIV, they truly brought to life every possible aspect.

In the episode "Howdy Partner" (S3 E13) Toni (Jill Marie Jones) is faced with the same situation as Samantha from *Sex and the City*, the fear common with needing to be tested. From the start Toni highlights the concern that Todd must think she is "dirty" for even suggesting they get tested, "Todd wants me to get an HIV Test. . . . For him to suggest I get one must mean that he thinks I have cooties or something." Offering a supportive and simple response Lynn replies, "Or he is smart. I get one every six months." Knowing the long-standing history of Lynn's past Toni continues to focus on the stereotype of who needs to be tested. "Yeah, but you need one, you're a whore. I mean before him it had been two years. If I had something I

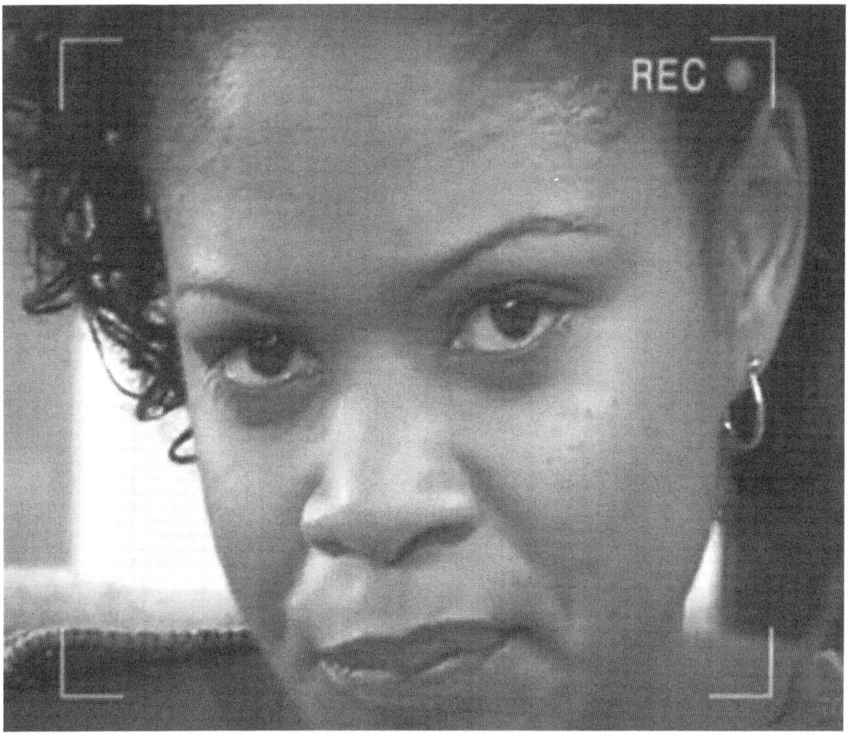

Figure 5.1. ***Girlfriends*, "Sex, Lies, and Books" (2003). Source: Paramount Network Television**

wouldn't look this healthy and fabulous." At this point Toni shifts into a second stereotype that one would know they are "sick" because symptoms would be present. Thankfully Lynn is again able to provide a voice of truth by informing Toni that a person can be asymptomatic for years and still have contracted the virus. Lynn then specifically asks Toni about her testing history,

Lynn: When was the last time you had an HIV test?

Toni: Look at me, I don't need that mess! (snaps) Obviously I'm blessed.

Lynn: You need to take this test.

Toni: . . . listen if I am going to die, I am going to do it ignorant and happy.

Lynn: No, you need to take this test. IF you have HIV (and I am sure you don't) you need to find out. You could pass it so someone you care about . . . and you don't have to die. ESP if you can catch it before you have symptoms. There are drugs now, people are living long lives with the virus.

Toni's remark about being "blessed" raises yet another common trope about testing: HIV and AIDS as punishment for poor behavior. Later when talking with another of the friends the notion of punishment is discussed directly, "Taking the test has made me think about what kind of person I am. I just want to make sure I am square with the lord. . . . Maya, I am really scared. I haven't always practiced safe sex. And I haven't always walked with Jesus. I'm telling you, Maya, getting the AIDS . . . it's going to be my punishment." Similarly, to only a handful of other shows, her friend Maya quickly retorts, "Toni . . . no one deserves AIDS. You are not a bad person." Again, offering support but also neglecting the real risk that unsafe sex comes with. In the end, Toni's results are negative; consistent with all the other situational comedies the character is redeemed of past indiscretions, and order in the show is restored.

In the previous examples female friends are observed having open and honest conversations about relationships, sex, and although occurring rarely, testing for STIs and HIV. For single women in their 20s and 30s such discussions should be commonplace. However, talking about STIs and HIV in the "golden" years of life offers an whole new perspective. As mentioned when discussing Saul's test in *Brothers and Sisters* older generations are one of the fastest growing populations of new HIV infections. Speaking directly to this audience the show *The Golden Girls* also included a narrative of HIV (S5 E19).

Receiving a letter from a hospital Rose, played by Betty White, is asked to come in for "a test." According to the letter the blood she received may have contained HIV antibodies; thus an informative and relatable narrative of HIV is presented. Throughout the episode Rose processes the need for the test and the possibility that she might have HIV; she begins to panic. Multiple times she states that she is scared, terrified, and worried about what will happen.

Continuing the theme of a character being "just fine" the audience observes the friends coming to the rescue with words of encouragement and the phrase "you will be just fine." Here, however, the phrase is simply mentioned and they move on to another topic. Later, however, Blanche (Rue McClanahan) reveals that she too has taken an HIV test given her lavish history with men. Blanche states that since taking the test she has changed her behaviors and now talks with her partners about their history and "we take all the necessary precautions." Blanche's disclosure that she openly talks with partners about testing and protection is encouraging and could have set a foundation for other shows to include such discussions; however, this is one of the few moments where such a conversation takes place.

Laying a foundation for other important conversations about HIV this episode also tackles many of the challenges those living with HIV face daily including abandonment and system-wide barriers. On the day of Rose's test her fears of being positive return to the conversation. "Well I might as well get used to doing things alone." Challenged on what she means, Rose continues: "Come on. If that tests turns out to be positive you're not going to want to be around me." Unlike the previous examples, Rose speaks directly to the fear of abandonment many faced during the early 80s. Without a clear understanding of how HIV was passed from person to person many living with the virus lost friends and family as soon as the results came in. Rose's fears thus echo the realities of that time including the fear of how she would ever tell her partner Myles. Thankfully, Rose has a support system that is able to calm her anxieties and provide reassurance that this is "just a test" and she will be "just fine." However, by focusing on these assurances there is a lack of discussion of what would happen if in fact she did have the virus. As Rose explains near the end of the episode the comments of "you will be fine" and "take it easy" are in fact not helpful at lowering the fear at all. What is needed is clear support and empathy. The statement you will be "just fine" for many of the shows implies empathy and support but what the characters, and audiences, need to hear is "we will be here no matter what." The promise to be a support no matter what would offer a more powerful and effective level of empathy than simply saying of course you will not have it. "Just fine" also leads a viewer to believe that those who are living with the virus are not "fine"; they are in some way broken.

During her checkin she is told that the hospital encourages anonymity so if she wanted to use a fake name she could. Rose does as she chooses her friend's name (a friend who is standing beside her). Though it might have been possible to receive anonymous testing at a hospital in the past, today this would not be the case. Sitting in the waiting room Rose says, "This is creepy, fake names?" Finally, speaking to the many challenges of living with HIV Blanche comments, "People who test positive cannot get insurance, lose jobs, it's terrible." Though brief, this acknowledgment of the challenge people living with the virus face is one of the few moments in the comedic genre to discuss the systemic barriers.

Speaking to the larger social issues surrounding HIV the show also includes a discussion of the lack of conversation parents have with teens about sex and HIV. Talking with her own mother, Dorothy (Bea Author) reads over a flier, lamenting that given how important the topic of HIV is, they (parents of teens) "should be able to get past their embarrassment." Remarking on how progressive she was as a mother, Sophia (Estelle Getty) comments on how open she was in talking about sex. Yet as Dorothy reveals, "Oh yes, Ma, I remember you using such technical terms. Don't let a boy touch your you know where." The fact that Sophia engaged in the conversation at all may have been progressive at the time, but the language used was clearly limited. The real moment of progress, though again not in terms of language, occurs, however, when Sophia tells Dorothy that given all that is happening she picked up some condoms (handing her a brown paper bag), explaining that the man needs to "put this on his you know where."

During the three days of waiting, viewers observe the emotional torture Rose experiences wondering what will happen. It is also during this time that Sophia also reveals her fear of HIV. Being questioned about why Sophia has been using Dorothy's bathroom she states, "because there is something wrong with mine. . . . Rose used it." Here again the show directly tackles the social stigma surrounding the topic at this time. Slightly condemning her mother, Dorothy exclaims, "Ma, that is just ignorant paranoia. It is attitudes like that that add to the panic of all this. What is wrong with you?" This scene touches on the fear and misperception common in the late 80s that HIV could be contracted from touching everyday items such as door handles, coffee cups, and toilet seats. Sophia explains that while she knows intellectually that she cannot catch get it, knowing it could be so close to home is scary. Scenes such as this should have been far more common, however, only a small handful of shows examined explicitly discussed the trepidation friends have with being around HIV.

The same year Rose's friends narrowly escaped HIV, another group of friends, this time college students, looked directly into the face of HIV through the eyes of a classmate. Building from the success of *The Cosby Show* a tight group of students could be found walking the halls of Hillman College, a fictional historically Black college in Virginia. Over the course of six seasons *A Different World* challenged viewers' perceptions of a number of heavy topics including date rape, classism, racism, equal rights, and in its third season HIV. In the episode "If I Should Die Before I Wake" (S4 E23), two crucial conversations occur, one on the topic of condom use and the other the realities of living with HIV.

During a public speaking class, students were required to give their own eulogies. When it is Josie's (Tisha Campbell-Martin) turn, the room quickly turns somber as she explains, ". . . by the following Spring, Josie had died from acquired immunodeficiency syndrome. The disease we all know as AIDS." In her speech she tells the class how she contracted the virus from having unprotected sex with her boyfriend, "He was smart, fun, all star quarterback. Neither of us knew he was HIV positive." Her words bring some in the room to tears, and others to questions.

Whitley: I don't. I, I, I don't understand. This is not a woman's disease.

Kim: Tell that to the 16 thousand women who have it.

Whitley: They use drugs. Or they do perverted things.

Professor: AIDS is NOT a moral judgment.

Whitley: How come she couldn't tell by looking at him?

Josie: Because you can tell by looking at me? Can you tell I'm dying?

Unlike any of the other comedic shows that took on the challenge of HIV this scene is the only one that did not incorporate a joke surrounding HIV. As a result, the mood of the scene remains serious and even tense. Ramping up the tension, another student in the class leans over to her friend to remark, "Girl, I live down the hall from that girl. I am going to have to switch dorms." Without missing a beat Kim replies with the fact that HIV is only transmitted through fluids. Finally, after an emotional six minutes, the scene is ruptured with a joke from a nerdy-looking young man explaining suddenly it's OK with him that he has never had sex.

MEN'S APPROACHES TO TALKING ABOUT HIV

One of the most interesting, and problematic, observations of how HIV has been covered in sitcoms is the difference in tone between men's and women's approaches to discussing the topic. While multiple conversations about HIV occurred between women of various ages and races, far fewer shows included men sharing in such dialogue. As discussed already this chapter, some sitcoms offered countless HIV prevention and testing messages, each targeting multiple social, political, and medical aspects of the illness. When it came to men talking about HIV, a significantly different approach was taken.

Returning to *A Different World* for a moment, a direct result of Josie's powerful speech is the inspiration for Dwayne (Kadeem Hardison) and his roommate Ron (Darryl Bell) to talk risk and consequences of their own behaviors. In a moment of Ron poking fun at Dwayne for having a "short list," the list of women he had slept with, Dwayne retorts, "Hey man, the shorter the list, the smaller the risk." Immediately Ron falls to the couch in exasperation. "I'm doomed! I tried to be responsible. You know how it is. You just get caught unprepared. And you say to yourself, hey it can't happen to me." The men's conversation is short lived, however, and ends with the plan for each to get tested. This unfortunately ends the examples of men talking about testing in sitcoms. Instead the men of comedy focus on the lighter sides of talking about HIV.

Take for instance the medical comedy *Scrubs*. In a 2009 episode, "My New Moon" (S8 E13), Dr. Reid (Sarah Chalke) is confronted with a patient whom she originally thinks is simply anorexic. When the blood work comes back the results show HIV, and Dr. Reid is faced with how to tell her patient. Confiding to a fellow doctor she is told: "Well, it might not be that bad. HIV isn't a death sentence anymore." During the conversation Dr. Turk (Donald Faison) tries to explain why HIV isn't that scary; he even alters the pronunciation (pronounced Hiv EE), "I heard someone else call it that, and it sounded cooler, something that could almost be a dance." At this point Turk begins to demonstrate the "doing the Hiv EE" dance. Confused only for a moment Dr. Reid gives Dr. Turk a questionable look, but soon joins in the movement.

While making HIV into a hip new dance move is less than appropriate, the manner through with two characters in FX's show *Always Sunny in Philadelphia* (S12 E2) discuss HIV is even more egregious. While waiting in line at a waterpark Frank (Danny DeVito) and Charlie (Charlie Day) discover a special program for kids with leukemia allowing them to go first. Not wanting to have to wait Frank begins screaming, "AIDS, I've got the AIDS," pushing through to the front of the line. Continuing his rant he says, "No, I'm not gay. There are two kinds of AIDS. There is the vagina AIDS and the needle-based AIDS. I have the vagina kind. All AIDS are bad. There is no good AIDS, but I am not the gay AIDS."

Frank and his friend take their "AIDS bit" so far as to put suction marks on Frank to sell the bit, "I even give him lesions by sucking on his chest." After running around the entire park screaming AIDS Frank gets a cut on his back, bleeding into the pool. Children who notice begin pointing and screaming, "Hey he has AIDS," as they run away.

Taking a similar approach, another FX show using HIV as a punchline was *The League*. In the 2013 season (S5 E1), Ted (Adam Brody) is introduced to the primary characters and is quickly outed for having "the AIDS." Not just HIV, but "full blownsies" AIDS. Disturbingly, the whole group raises glasses of champagne and energetically toasts "to AIDS!"

As everyone swigs their champagne, Ted smiles and says, "I drank out of all those glasses." A few hesitate, one character spits out the champagne before he declares it a joke. As the final friend, Rafi (Jason Mantzoukas), arrives Ted is once again introduced as "and this is Ted, he has AIDS." Without missing a beat Rafi offers some advice: "Dude, what you do is, every day take a baby aspirin. If you need to fly take two. I swear. You do that and that shit will clear up in a month."

Throughout the four episodes Ted is seen, he continues to provide "hilarity" by pretending to cut himself, and showing people how great it is to live with AIDS. In one scene, a particularly dumb friend decides the success Ted is experiencing in life must be because his HIV cocktail makes him smart. To test this theory he steals Ted's medication, swallows a day's worth, and gains the pleasure of explosive diarrhea.

As crass and crude as the show is during a normal episode, the jokes surrounding Ted's AIDS push the lines of what comedy is in a number of ways. When the show's producer Jeff Schaffer was asked about the storylines he explained

> This isn't a pity story; it's a jealousy story. We get to play with something you usually don't see a lot in comedy—people's discomfort around AIDS and someone who has AIDS, all of the miseducation about how you get it, and when it's contagious, and all that kind of stuff. But that comedy only lasts for a beat. Then the real fun for us was that these guys are jealous of him. They're jealous of his AIDS. They're jealous of his life.

Even the character Kevin (Stephen Rannazzisi) is heard saying at one point "Full-blown Ted has a better life than I do. I want to be like that guy. I want to be the guy with AIDS."

In each of the episodes from *The League* and *Always Sunny in Philadelphia* characters are seen and heard remarking they want to be like those living with the virus. For viewers of these shows, not only is the lesson that HIV is no big deal, but even better, it's desirable. Admittedly, viewers of these shows know the conversation surrounding HIV are jokes. However, these are missing vital opportunities to even mention facts about risks. Instead they choose to fully focus on framing HIV as a joke.

Although most of the men in the episodes use HIV as a vehicle to get what they want, one episode allowed for a male character to take a political stand providing a platform for people to talk about and consider social issues. Following in the footsteps of comedians across the globe an episode of *Seinfeld* titled "The Ribbon" (S7 E9) bridges a gap of making a social statement and a joke. Airing in 1995, the episode shows Kramer (Michael Richards) walking in solidarity for a local charity AIDS Walk. What makes him stand out, however, is his refusal to wear an AIDS ribbon during the walk.

Inspired by the real-life situation of a former *Days of Our Lives* actress Deidre Hall, who publicly refused to wear AIDS ribbons at public events. Upsetting many, the idea of "ribbon bullies," people pushing others to wear the ribbon to visually show support, was not far from reality. In a 1993 *Newsweek* article titled "Tyranny of the Red Ribbon," an HIV-positive photographer was interviewed about his take on the use of the AIDS ribbon, "It was revolting," he says. "I felt like I was being packaged into a neat little cause for people to pander to."

For Kramer, the resistance to wearing the ribbon begins with a number of people badgering him to wear the ribbon. Being handed the ribbon at the sign in he explains, "Oh no, I don't need one." Shocked, the woman at the table states, "But you *have* to wear the ribbon." When Kramer again refuses she is heard calling out, "Hey, get back here and put this on." While walking, yet another person asks him where his ribbon is. "Oh, I don't wear one." Quickly, those around him begin to question, "Aren't you against AIDS?" Trying to explain Kramer states, "Yes, I am against AIDS, I'm walking, aren't I? I just don't wear the ribbon." Not liking this answer, one lady challenges, "Who do you think you are" while another man yells out to some friends farther in the walk. Getting the attention of many angry walkers the scene ends with Kramer being chased down the street, cornering him near a fire escape, "SO, are you going to wear the ribbon? I am wearing the ribbon, he wears the ribbon, WE ALL wear the ribbon. Why don't you wear the ribbon?" Still standing his ground Kramer explains, "This is America. I don't have to wear anything I don't want to." As a result, the angry mob closes in and says, "Well I guess we'll just have to teach him to wear the ribbon." Trying to escape, he reaches for the fire escape ladder, but Kramer is pulled down and surrounded as the scene fades away.

Kramer's fight against having to visibly show support speaks to the early start of HIV apathy in the media. Additionally, the late 90s was also the start of new medications and treatments found to be effective; thus the death sentence was lifted. As a result, show writers may have found it appropriate to include jokes about HIV—a point which is clear when considering the steady decline of shows which would continue to talk about HIV and the increase of sarcasm found within the tone of nearly all future comedic narratives.

SATIRE AND SASS: HIV IN ANIMATED COMEDIES

Joining in on the joke, and possibly sparking some of the initial flames, animated comedies have also taken on the topic of HIV in crude and boundary-pushing ways. Pushing the limits on nearly every topic it was no shock to see *South Park* taking on the topic. Incorporating a spoof of the movie *Philadelphia*, to claiming Magic Johnson was cured by drinking a blended concoction of money, the creators provide yet another message to viewers that HIV is so normal that now it can be the center of a joke. To this point one scene in the series even explains that "After 22.2 years, it's official. AIDS is finally funny!" (S12 E1). With the words spoken the town rejoices, celebrating with streamers and confetti and the new statue in the town reveals the same message.

Unlike *South Park* each of the other animated HIV moments were far less of the central focus of an episode. Offering an explanation as to where HIV originated, *Family Guy* creator Seth MacFarlane created a short clip titled "The Creation of Aids." Opening with a black screen with white words the viewer reads: "Several years ago a rumor began that the first human ever 'patient zero' to contract AIDS had been identified. He was a gay Canadian flight attendant. Here is his story." In the following minutes viewers observe a man and a monkey waiting at the airport. After a few seconds it becomes clear that the man is "hitting on" the monkey. The man asks if the monkey comes to the States often, but when he discovers this is not the case he simply asks, "So you want to just have sex now then?" To which the monkey replies, "Now you're talking," and jumps on top of the guy as they begin to kiss. In the next scene, the two are in bed with the monkey on top thrusting away. At the end of their session, the man tells the monkey, "So I guess I should tell you. I kinda have this disease that makes your immune system kinda go away. Other than that, I am clean as a whistle." Seeing that the monkey is not concerned, the conversation continues.

Man: Hey, thanks for not making me use a condom.

Monkey: Oh, yeah no problem.

Man: Wanna go again?

Monkey: Let's pound it, brother!

Although the scene mostly seems ridiculous, it is one of the only narratives to address one of the many ideas about the origins of HIV. There have been conspiracies surrounding the idea that HIV came from monkeys; this clip offers the "humor" in the notion that HIV was indeed passed from sex with a monkey but flips the script and blames the human. Toeing the line of funny and outright offensive, multiple critics and fans called the show out for going too far.

Focusing on another stereotype in an animated series, yet again by MacFarlane, *American Dad* creates a moment with Rodger, an alien, who has contracted HIV from prison. Explaining why he is planning to reform his ways he says, "Now that I have been raped by some guys who actually know what they are doing, I just want to share. You know, give a little back" (S8 E11). Assuming he means his money, Hayley (voiced by Rachael MacFarlane) asks if he will give all his money away but is hit in the throat and is not able to finish the question. Rodger replies, "I am sorry dear, I couldn't hear you. My ears are not working so well. I got AIDS in prison. (long pause, and seeing questioning faces) Hearing Aids. I really should keep them in. Then I would have heard that guy when he snuck up on me in the shower and gave me HIV." Aside from the punchline of his joke, HIV nor AIDS is ever mentioned again in the show.

In writing for these shows MacFarlane repeatedly presents only quick mentions of HIV. In each spot social criticism, stereotypes, and satire is implemented. The concern, however, is that only those with deeper understanding of the issues being addressed are likely to understand the "joke." Without understanding the truth or history of the comments it is likely the viewers will take the messages only at face value: learning that AIDS came from monkeys, with enough money you can cure HIV, and that indeed HIV is finally funny.

STANDING UP WITH HIV

Taking the jokes on the road some stand-up comedians have joined in on commenting about HIV. Similar to the jokes made in the animated comedies and shows on FX many of the jokes are pointed directly at the virus. Also consistent is the use of the idea of "full blown" AIDS. One such example, although not one of her stand-up bits, occurred in an Amy Schumer sketch for Comedy Central. In the scene Amy is having a lovely date with a man she seems to have been dating for a short while. Planning for later evening events her date informs her that he has AIDS. Initially Amy pretends she didn't hear him, but quickly states that it's fine, "It's not a deal breaker at all." A bit surprised, her date sits back in his chair and smiles. As the conversation continues Amy asks about the "kind of AIDS" her date has, asking if it is HIV. The date tries a few times to explain that, no, he in fact has AIDS and not HIV. Appearing to finally understand, Amy moves on and thanks her date for his honesty and attempts to show she is just fine with his status, "Ummm. I am ok. Actually, I think I really am. I'm sorry. I just had a moment. I mean people do this. If we just use protection, and you know don't share needles. We should be fine. . . . I think it's kinda cool. you know kinda badass. It's like the 90s are back. Do you go to a lot of events?" To which the date retorts, "No, I go to a lot of doctors." Amy's line of questions and awkward pauses are both understandable and typical for many people who might be told their date has an illness such as HIV or AIDS. And while there are a few moments for a punchline to occur, the real joke is heard when her date discovers that Amy has a gluten allergy, "Oh I can't have that. I have a gluten allergy, so that torte would be like my AIDS." Watching as her date gets up she asks if he needs to take care of some AIDS-related complication, "Full disclosure I didn't see *Philadelphia*, but I did see *Gia*, so I feel fully prepared to help." Showing signs of annoyance, the date gathers his things and states, "No, I'm leaving. I'm sorry I am a total foodie, and I think gluten allergies are just bull." The scene depicts an important challenge for anyone living with HIV, choosing if and when to disclose their status. At first the conversation seems to fit the uneasiness both parties are likely to feel. However, the choice to focus so much time on the "full blown AIDS" aspect is both unrealistic and more awkward than funny.

Also offering a far more awkward moment of comedy is part of a Dave Chappelle stand-up routine (*Block Party*, 2005) in which he discusses the origins of AIDS. Taking a page from the *Family Guy* playbook Dave only addresses the idea that AIDS came from a monkey.

> I don't know where it came from. No one knows where AIDS came from. Scientists say AIDS came from when a man had sex with a monkey. [makes disgusted face] Word? After all this research this is the best you can come up with? Nobody f*cks monkeys and people, you idiot. You either f*ck monkeys. Or you f*ck people. That's it. There is no in between.

The bit continues to graphically describe the process of courting and having sex with a monkey, but never mentions AIDS again. Luckily, many of the other examples found where HIV was incorporated into a stand-up bit did provide some level of education or at the very least made direct strides toward raising social awareness.

Addressing the ignorance others still have about the virus Comedy Central newcomer Trevor Noah shared a conversation he had with a young surfer girl in California upon hearing he is from South Africa (Comedy Central Special, *That's Racist*, 2013).

> Surfer Girl: SO if you are like from Africa, have you like ever had AIDS?
>
> Trevor: So you know what is funny. I wasn't offended that she said AIDS. What I was offended by is that she said *had* AIDS, like it was something you could ever have had. Like a passing flu. (Makes another joke about people having a bit of the AIDS, but now I'm better.) Ever had AIDs. Now I know, I know as a child of a continent that has been ravaged by an illness that it is my job, my duty, to educate people whenever I can. But you know when you meet someone and you look into their eyes and you know . . . there's no hope. There is only two of us, and I am bored so why not have some fun. So I say yes. Yes I have had the AIDS many many times.
>
> Surfer Girl: OMG REALLY. WOW Oh my God. So shouldn't you be like super skinny and dead or something?
>
> Trevor: Oh no, no, no. AIDS isn't as bad as you think. It's just like chocolate. You just don't want to have too much at one time. You have too much you feel bad, and then you feel better. You should try it sometime.
>
> Surfer Girl: NOOO, that's disgusting. If it's like chocolate it will be all melty and I'll get dirty.

Trevor: No, but then you just take a shower, and it washes right off.

Trevor's bit while poking direct fun at the young woman, highlights the fact that many people still think it is happening to the people in Africa, not to mention being oblivious to how HIV works. Specifically, the ideas of "had AIDS," and that people with the virus would only look like the stereotypes shown on television and movies, is discussed further in chapter seven. This conversation also makes note of the idea that HIV makes someone dirty. Noah's response to "washing the AIDS off" for many will be played off as being the joke, however, the deeper meaning of this line actually relates to the president of his country who had recently remarked about washing illnesses off of people.

The only real theme found within HIV stand-up comedy are the jokes about testing. Providing the earliest example is Chris Rock's *Bigger and Blacker* special aired in 1992.

He begins by relating the notion of taking the AIDS test to something you pass or fail. "I got the AIDS test. Passed it, got a 65." While a 65 would barely be considered a passing grade the joke is really a jab to the judgment surrounding the idea of "failing the test" and becoming HIV positive. Rock continues his discussion about the testing experience directing attention to what is really the most terrifying aspect, "What's scary about the AIDS test? What's scary is that you don't get the results for five days. What happens during that time? You start reflecting. You think back to every nasty ass, questionable piece of sex you ever had. And everybody got a few." Though the joke is short and to the point it actually does accurately identify the real problem with the original form of the test. Results of HIV tests in those days had to be sent to a city lab for processing and took on average three to five days. Thankfully testing has advanced dramatically and today only a tiny amount of blood is required, and is processed at the clinic while you wait about 20 minutes. That is unless you are Baron Vaughn.

In Vaughn's comedy routine he sets up the joke well by, for the first time in the idea of getting testing together, "we did the responsible thing, we got tested for all the stuff." He then continues to explain the process: "And they have this test now that can tell you in just 20 minutes. if you have HIV. Which I guess is just dandy." The story continues that his girlfriend is taken back for her test, then he is taken back 10 minutes later. This is where the pretest interview takes place, "They give you this sexual history interview. It's like a job interview for not being a whore." Returning from his interview his girlfriend is soon taken back and given her results, indicating that it should only be about 10 more minutes for his results to come back. After two hours pass by he begins to wonder, did they forget about him or are they "really, I mean really looking at my blood" or the possibility comes to his mind that "they are drawing straws to see who gets to give me the bad news."

Finally, he asks the woman at the desk and he is taken back to the far room, "When the lady comes in she puts her hand on my knee, looks at me concerned and says, 'I am so, so sorry. I went to lunch. You do not have HIV, but the ham and cheese sandwiches are delicious." For Vaughn, and I am sure anyone else who has had similar experiences, the stress of not knowing why the results are taking so long ignites a deep fear of what might be happening. Luckily, if this routine had been seen or joke had been shared, a small amount of ease is possible.

Finally, Sean Patton speaks directly to the audience about testing. Only for Patton the audience is not those who would be seeking testing to discover their status; instead he focuses on those who already know they are HIV positive.

> Is anyone here HIV positive? If you are laughing, don't feel bad. You know what does nothing for HIV, your sadness. If you are HIV + I am sorry that happened to you, but now I think you have just earned the right to be a perpetual prankster. You should have a fake blood dispenser on you at all times. Just ready to go. Ready to hose down anyone at bars or cops. "Oh my AIDS blood! It got everywhere." Or better yet, go to every clinic and get tested just to mess with the people.

As the joke continues he describes the multiple ways one could respond to the news. Including freaking out by screaming, crying hysterically, laughing like a clown, or turning into a robot. Though the ways in which people respond to a positive test result will vary, it is not uncommon for many of these situations to come to life, minus the clown or malfunctioning robot.

The only comedian to provide any type of facts about HIV, although again only calling it AIDS, was Donald Glover (*Weirdo*, 2011). Discussing why children are absolutely the worst Glover states, "that's why I wear condoms. I know some people say they wear condoms so they don't get AIDS. But I got to be honest. I'd rather get AIDS, than have a baby." He continues to make the point that when you really think about it there is little difference between the two,

> They are both expensive, both last the rest of your life, both remind you of the mistakes you made in the past, and once you have it you can pretty much only date other people who have it. What's the difference? The only difference is you can't go to jail for accidentally dropping AIDS. At least when people have AIDS, and others are aware they feel sorry for you. People want to help you out. People don't give a sh*t when you have kids.

To his point there are indeed these overlaps, although I am certain many parents would not compare their kids to an illness. At the same time, encouraging audience members to have protected sex as a means of avoiding these realities is not a bad approach.

DECADES OF COMEDY: WHAT HAVE WE BEEN LAUGHING AT?

Looking across the HIV narratives found within the comedic genre it became clear that the treatment of the topic was far less about the type of subgrene (sitcom, sketch, satire, cartoon, or stand-up) but far more dependent on the time frame and frames used by other mediums. The 80s focusing mostly on dispelling myths and raising awareness, the 90s emphasizing the need for testing while also attempting to break down continued stereotypes, and the 2000s centering on life with the illness. Finally, it is within the last eight years that HIV has become a common occurrence as a punchline within television shows. These larger themes illustrate how the HIV narrative has evolved from messages about confronting fear and stigma to just a chronic illness, just taboo enough to get a laugh. They also mirror the ways in which HIV and AIDS were being discussed in the times of which the shows aired.

In the 80s, HIV in a comedy was primarily used as a vehicle for prompting a larger discussion and raising awareness. HIV, the virus itself, was never the punchline. That is except for an awkward moment and quick one liner in a 1986 episode of *Mr. Belvedere* (S2 E16). Danny, played by Ian Fried, is introduced as a classmate and friend of the Owens' youngest child Wesley. After a series of scenes discussing Danny's AIDS status, the fear is of Wesley's "risk" of contracting AIDS given that the boys often talk on the phone and play together. Later in the show Danny comes to the house. Upon entering, the family asks how Danny is doing. To which he nonchalantly replies, "Well, I've got AIDS, but other than that I'm doing pretty good." Not sure what to say the parents simply look at each other and shrug. Refusing to see Danny, it becomes clear that Wesley is confused as to what AIDS is, and how people get it. Thankfully, the show takes the time to include in the family's conversation the facts, ending with Mr. Belvedere himself speaking to the classroom, and helps the kids move past their fears.

The quick joke about AIDS in *Mr. Belvedere* not only provided audience members the opportunity to observe how awkward it might be to find out someone you know is positive, but the fact it was a child who brought up the conversation allowed for less judgment. Danny's infection was not possibly his fault, and therefore could be used as a vehicle for open conversation about risk. This was also a reflection of the fact that it wasn't until Ryan White, a young person who had contracted the AIDS virus through a blood transfusion (thus, of no fault of his own), had come into the attention of the media that people as a whole could consider AIDS as anything beyond an illness infecting the gay population.

Shows such as *Designing Women*, *Golden Girls*, and *A Different World* also took on roles of challenging the social narratives and misperceptions being spread by the news media and people in general. These shows, as well as others examined, used the specific words commonly heard at the time, twisting them in such a way that it is almost impossible to think the statement or behavior would be appropriate. These shows highlighted the ridiculousness of thinking you could catch HIV from a coffee mug while also stating time and time again that HIV was not a punishment. It is the repetition of these messages across shows that had the greatest impact. Had only *Designing Women* challenged the notion of AIDS as a gay disease many might still to this day believe that is the case. Given that so many shows joined in the fight a shared narrative was created and multiple audiences were given the opportunity to hear facts about the virus.

Unfortunately, as medical advances improved and people began to feel apathetic about the topic of HIV the drive and interest waned. Fewer and fewer shows now feel the need to include HIV as a topic for means of raising awareness. However, even if the goal is not to stir up a social movement, small moments in a show can have a larger impact. Thus, any show including the topic of a preventable and stigmatized illness such as HIV must carefully consider the impact it could have. As mentioned in the show *Scrubs* we have to handle this better, "Don't try and make this OK. This is not OK. This is the worst thing that is ever going to happen to me in my entire life, and you are here to see it. So, you need to find a way to handle it better. I get to handle it however I want" (*Scrubs* S9 E13). For the doctors in the show, and for many viewers, HIV might not be seen as the big deal it was in the 80s and 90s, but for those living with the virus an HIV diagnosis is still life altering. Therefore, the notion of trying to find "cooler" ways to say HIV, or making it into a dance move might be funny for some; the show directly acknowledges that HIV is not really a laughing matter.

FRAMING HIV AS COMEDY

Having provided insight into how HIV has been presented within the comedic realm let us shift to the deeper lessons gained from these shows, considering why a comedic frame might be done in the first place. In the previous chapter, HIV and AIDS was presented through what rhetorical scholar Kenneth Burke refers to as the tragic frame.[2] Within a tragedy, the "evil" or wrongdoing is placed on the shoulders of a scapegoat. Within dramatic narratives the scapegoat is a secondary character that engaged in risky behavior beyond the knowledge of the central character. As was the case for any character whose past caught up to them. For more than 60 percent of the dramas examined the tragic frame could be applied. The character either engaged in an "immoral" risky behavior on screen, or in the past, and HIV was shown as the big punishment for those "crimes." In each of the cases the tragic frame blames and punishes the character, thus teaching the larger lesson, thus restoring the social order. Employing fear and shame, tragic framing often propels the same negative thoughts and feelings it seeks to dispel.

To remedy this paradox, television writers have discovered methods of writing HIV narratives into shows that allow for viewers to observe the poor choices, thus teaching a lesson, and correcting the behavior without the use of punishment or shaming. These lessons occur by putting Burke's comic frame into practice. The goal of the comic frame is not to mortify the character, or in this case stigmatize those who are HIV positive. Instead the comic frame seeks to "teach the fool—and vicariously the audience—about error so that it may be corrected rather than punished" (Brummett 1984, 220). Doing so allows for the character, and viewer, to learn an important lesson while still remaining part of the larger community.

By implementing the comic frame, shows can present lessons of the inappropriateness of promiscuous sex, or drug use, while also maintaining a sense of shared community, allowing for the parasocial relationships to remain intact while also teaching the viewer that the offender can be reformed. The character might feel guilt for their behavior, however, they will be able to overcome this guilt by talking to other characters including family, peers, and/or medical providers. Once "reformed" the character is able to come back to the community, thus maintaining the social order.

Applying Burke's ideas to HIV narratives across comedic shows provides insight into the dilemmas and paradoxes associated with including serious health issues as punchlines. When shows successfully invoke a comedic frame, observers not only see the implications of their actions, they also learn it is acceptable to make mistakes. However, with mistakes should come serious consequences.

But Is HIV Funny??

When examining the number of HIV narratives within dramas over the years a steady decline is discovered. Looking at the rates of HIV narratives within comedies the opposite is true. In some ways this reversal is explained by the sheer fact that HIV/AIDS is no longer a death sentence, and is far less mysterious than it was in the 80s and 90s. However, it is still life altering and deeply stigmatized. Thus, for a personal friend Danny and others who live with the virus, "there is NOTHING funny about HIV."

During the course of researching HIV and advocating for sexual health education I have had the pleasure of working closely with countless inspiring men and women who live with the virus. While collecting shows for this chapter I took the opportunity to reconnect with a few of these friends and the topic of HIV as a punchline came up. I admitted that personally I struggled to ever find humor in the jokes being told, but I wanted to know their feelings. Resoundingly the answer was the same, "It really pisses me off," Danny stated. "There is still WAY too much stigma involved." Another friend commented that for those who have lived with the illness for a while it is possible to see the humor, however, for those who are newly diagnosed these jokes only poor salt in the already painful wounds.

Though some levity can help normalize a difficult conversation, using comedy to educate audiences about a serious illness creates a very thin line for writers to walk. Not surprisingly, the best examples of comedic HIV narratives were found in the shows where writers worked with outside sources to craft an engaging and informative show. *Girlfriends* and *A Different World* each provide scripts of how friends can talk to each other about condom use, testing, even living with the virus. Viewers not only acquire facts about testing, they also observe positive experiences. This said, the fact is that not all writers are including HIV into the storyline for the purpose of education.

Taking the social media posts of *Family Guy* creator Seth MacFarlane into account it would be difficult to argue he has any goal of raising awareness about HIV. Instead the primary focus is on gaining the laugh. Drawing from misperceptions, popular myths, and possibly the jokes of others his skits do nothing for the viewer beyond enforcing the idea that HIV is an immoral act. Even when a barbershop quartet is used to tell a patient he has "the AIDS" not "HIV, but full blown AIDS," messages of judgment are apparent when they sing "you might have gotten it from when you put that filthy needle in here" pointing to the patient's arm "or from all that unprotected sex we hear." Each joke whether sung or written paints HIV in a light that only enforces that HIV is no big deal. When combined with the fact that fewer news reports or general mentions of HIV are present in today's narratives, if the only mention is in the form of a joke the audience's perceptions are likely to become limited.

NOTES

1. Interview with the writer. http://www.glaad.org/blog/linda-bloodworth-thomason-talks-glaad-about-bridegroom-designing-women-and-using-tv-social.
2. Kenneth Burke. *Attitudes toward history*. Berkeley: University of California Press, 1984.

Chapter Six

Didactic Dichotomy of HIV Narratives

The analysis of over three decades of episodes made it apparent that HIV has been represented within a very rigid dichotomy: normalized versus stigmatized. On one hand narratives highlight various groups talking about the issue of HIV over coffee or with friends and family. Using phrases such as "It's normal," "everyone should be tested," "I test all the time," and "It's like spring cleaning," frames the topic of testing for HIV as something everyone does. As a result, viewers are able to witness that conversations about sexually related topics are not taboo or difficult to discuss. Conversely, remarks about "the AIDS," "it's nasty," and "it will be my punishment" frame HIV as something to be feared and avoided. Thus, encouraging stigma and discrimination of people living with HIV.

Within most of the narratives viewers are provided facts about HIV while observing a myriad of emotions. Each show allowing the audience to witness how HIV conversations can occur, providing a potential script to be mirrored later. The lessons presented in the shows were overwhelmingly quite simple: get tested, talk to your partner (and friends) about getting tested, use condoms, and, though only mildly emphasized, everyone should consider their risk. Looking across the decades and genres, however, more complicated lesson are identified. Expanding out to a macro level of analysis common themes within the overall narrative structure of the shows as well as the language used when discussing the topic of HIV arc presented.

THE NARRATIVE STRUCTURES

To examine the structure of a narrative, one must look at how elements are working together to reveal the theme. Structure includes both the order and the unity of events or topics. At the most fundamental level, order can refer to having a clear beginning, middle, and end. For any show where the lesson is to encourage testing, this plot structure begins with the threat of HIV. The threat commonly arrives in the form of a foil[1] character, typically a current or previous sexual partner. The middle scenes center on choosing if the primary character will get tested, the test itself, and the process of waiting. It is during this section that the internal conflict is observable. Finally, the test results are discovered. Thus, providing relief for most, but also devastation for some. Episodes with other lessons, highlighting what it is like to live with the virus, for instance, the structure still begins with confusion about risk for HIV. An HIV-positive character discloses their status to the immediate shock, sadness, and confusion of those in the room. Throughout the show misperceptions are dispelled with facts, and in the end, all involved are wiser, and those living with the virus are given the vital support they need.

Following a week to week structural order, shows strive to have each story wrapped up in short, one- to two-week packages, allowing for new viewers to join in at any point. However, Sillars and Gronbeck (2001) argue that repeated formulaic order eliminates the potential for discovery. In other words, if the viewer is able to predict the ending, given the history with the show, then they may be less likely to completely engage and allow themselves to become involved. Therefore, if the structure used to present HIV is formulaic, it may eliminate the ability for audiences to make connections to their own lives. Unfortunately for HIV prevention, this concern of formulaic structure is at play.

The Redemption Narrative

The most dominant structure found within the episodes follows what Burke calls a redemptive narrative. This structure occurs in nearly every episode, aired after 1995, where a main character is first confronted with the need to test for HIV (i.e., *Golden Girls*, *Nip/Tuck*, *Girlfriends*, *Sex and the City*). This confrontation typically transpires when a past lover returns announcing that they have HIV. These secondary characters are frequently only included in one or two episodes and used simply to offer localized complication and drama. As a result, the main character is overwhelmed with "what ifs," and a fear that HIV will be the punishment for past behaviors takes form. One example of this is when the character Toni states, "I'm telling you, Maya, getting the AIDS. . . . It's going to be my punishment" (*Girlfriends*, S3 E13). Ultimately, however, each of the characters is redeemed by a negative HIV test and order is returned. By utilizing such a structure, risky behavior is represented as inconsequential. As a result, the viewer, especially if identifying with the character and situations, may feel less vulnerable to such consequences and therefore may not feel the need for HIV testing or behavioral change.

This redemptive structure appeared in a number of shows all sharing a happily ever after ending. That is unless the central character was gay. When both Saul, *Brothers and Sisters*, and Oliver, *How to Get Away with Murder*, seek testing each discover they are in fact HIV-positive. Thus, not offered the same redemption over a dozen straight charters were given. While statistically speaking the ratio of people tested on television to those receiving a positive test may be similar, and it is true certain populations are at greater risk, by only showing gay characters testing positive, stereotypes and a false sense of security become perpetuated.

Given this consistent structure, viewers are repeatedly observing that straight, young, white characters do not contract the virus. Thus, the manner through which HIV has been presented may ultimately teach young viewers that they do not have to be concerned about their own risk, given that characters that look like them are rarely shown impacted by HIV. However, for viewers who are gay, or African American women, HIV is in fact a concern. The notion of being redeemed by the end of the show, however, is far more than simply receiving a negative test. The direct language of HIV being a punishment, and then seeing only certain groups of people contracting the virus, reaffirms the long-standing fears that began in the 80s.

HIV as Punishment

Describing any illness as a punishment instills an idea that having an illness is shameful. Thus, increasing a sense of internalized stigma and guilt. Given the manner through which HIV was discussed from the beginning it is no surprise that the mediated narratives began echoing the social conversation. What was surprising is that the punishment narrative in the 80s and early 90s was dominantly about dispelling the idea that HIV was a punishment. Ninety percent of episodes included the line of dialogue, but it was the earliest episodes that offered an immediate counternarrative. Shows such as *Designing Women*, *Golden Girls*, *Life Goes On*, and *A Different World* each included discussion about how HIV not only impacts everyone, but each spoke directly that HIV was in no way a punishment. The episode of *Golden Girls* (S5 E19) provides one of the clearest examples. Finally reaching a breaking point while waiting for her test results Rose lashes out at Blanche stating, "This isn't supposed to happen to people like me. You must have gone to bed with hundreds of men. All I had was one innocent operation." Feeling hurt, Blanche challenges, asking if Rose thinks that it should be her. Rose explains, "No. I just mean I am a good person." With a sigh, Blanche reaches out to Rose and calmly reminds her that "AIDS is not a bad person's disease. It is not God punishing people for their sins."

Up to even the most modern HIV narratives, the phrase "it will be my punishment" is used. Disturbingly, the counternarrative that was common in the earlier episodes is rarely found post 2000. In the few places where a character is heard offering assurance, the focus is not on how HIV isn't a punishment, but instead the conversation shifts the focus to "you will be ok" and "YOU don't have HIV." These forms of assurances are then reaffirmed by the socially accepted characters receiving a negative test. In contrast, the characters that fit the "profile" of the highest rates of HIV populations hear no mention of "you'll be fine." The punishment narrative is then reinforced when they receive an HIV-positive test.

The contradicting narratives of everyone is at risk, yet only certain types of characters will be punished, furthers the myth that only some populations contract HIV. As a result, fear of the virus, and being perceived as someone who could have the virus, is perpetuated. Beyond perceptions of fear, young straight viewers are also exposed to lessons that HIV is not a consequence for their own sexual behavior. Therefore, testing would not be needed and condoms would only be required as means of preventing the only real punishment, teen pregnancy.

Drama and Guilt

Another component of nearly every HIV storyline was the narrative theme of guilt. Cutting across decades, genres, and subgenres numerous characters visually and verbally expressed feelings of guilt. The term "guilt" covers a variety of feelings including; tension, anxiety, shame, disgust, embarrassment, etc. Burke argues that it is through public discourse that ultimately motivates a person to work through feelings of guilt. Thus, guilt redemption is considered the plot of all human drama, and the means of maintaining social order.

Burke argues that guilt is inherent in all societies because people cannot accept all of the demands traditional hierarchy places on them. Moreover, even though American society is reliant on the use of sex to sell movies, books, and cars, engaging in sexual behavior for anything beyond procreation is taboo and shameful. Therefore, to maintain social order populations must be taught lessons about hierarchy and proper behaviors. Applying Burke's dramatistic process, social order is taught through a three-step cycle. First is the push against order (or hierarchy). In the cases of HIV narratives this is the moment characters engage in behaviors that are not of "high moral stature." Discovering their actions have consequences, the fear that HIV will be a punishment, the second stage of feeling guilt is achieved. Whenever a person rejects the traditional hierarchy, a feeling of failure is imminent and, consequently, the person will begin to feel a sense of guilt.

To keep order, characters that are still fitting social norms, not using drugs or gay, can still be spared. They are shown worried and guilt ridden, but in the end, redemption is possible. If, however, the character is not fitting into the social norms, they cannot be saved and redemption is not possible given there must be examples of why actions are not encouraged. These characters are therefore the victims, even scapegoats, used to mortify people into proper behavior.

Understanding that people were already condemning people with HIV, shows in the 80s and early 90s attempted to challenge the redemption narrative. Speaking directly to the perception that HIV was "killing all the right people," as stated in *Designing Women*. These early shows also included a wider variety of characters contracting the virus. In fact, more straight characters were shown contacting HIV in the 90s than any other population. However, these characters were in some ways redeemed, as few were shown experiencing the final days of the AIDS death. The same could not be said for the gay characters. Many of the characters shown sick and dying of the virus had contracted the virus from drug use or anal sex. Thus, the lesson to support social norms was still presented.

HIV to Punish

Following alongside the narrative of HIV being a punishment was an only slightly different narrative of HIV as a means of punishing others. Across the decades many of the legal/crime procedural shows depicted HIV as a method for others to punish those they felt were doing wrong. In most shows the HIV as punishment narrative followed a storyline of infected men purposely seeking out anyone who would be foolish enough to sleep with them, "if they are not smart enough to insist on a condom, they are getting what they deserve" (*CSI: New York* S3 E16). These characters often disclosed later they felt alone or hurt by the person who had given the virus to them, and by infecting others the pain and frustration would be shared.

Taking the framework of HIV as punishment to a whole new level was HBO's *OZ*. Launching headfirst into this idea an inmate is forced to work on the AIDS floor. After fighting with an inmate, Miguel Alvarez, Kirk Acevedo, is sent to the AIDS floor as a means of gaining some level of compassion, and to help reduce his overwhelming homophobia. Hearing this is where he is being sent Alvarez states "AIDs is what they get for being fags" (*Oz* S1 E1). After witnessing firsthand the living hell that was AIDS Alvarez, arguably, does appear to gain a new perspective.

Providing a graphic and more violent narrative, HIV as punishment was also found as inmates working on the AIDS floor acquired infected blood as a tool for infecting inmates in the other areas of the prison. In another episode an inmate, knowing he is HIV positive, persists on raping fellow inmates, or cutting himself and others. Finally, after identifying the "punishment" of having to work on the AIDS floor, yet another inmate acts out in order to be sent. Once there he steals a needle from the nurses station and proceeds to infect himself with the virus. Upon confirming his diagnosis, he sets to making other inmates his "sex slave." Within each of these situations little remorse or guilt is ever shown unless the character is in the final stages of the illness and finally facing death.

THE LANGUAGES OF HIV

Showing one group as victim or scapegoat and another as worthy of redemption is only one way social order is maintained. Another is the tone used when talking about behaviors or topics related to the behavior. One of the most interesting, and yet unsettling, themes found in watching 35 years of HIV television narratives is the strategic use of HIV or AIDS.

In the beginning of the epidemic the phrases of "gay cancer" or "gay plague" were understandable, although deeply damaging. It was not clear what was happening or the cause. When the name AIDS was coined it was again the language of the time and situation. Those three letters themselves filled people with fear and uncertainty. By the time HIV was identified there was still questions and fear, however, each day more knowledge was being gained and medications were starting to be developed. Decades later the general public, at least on a basic level, now understands that HIV causes AIDS, and that it is transmitted through bodily fluids. Few people today die of HIV, and when medication is taken, even fewer ever develop AIDS. Though, even with these realities the use of AIDS in television narratives remains staggering.

Regardless of genre both HIV and AIDS are heard within the narratives. While the average person might use them interchangeably, the connotation in many of the shows did not imply equal meaning. Overwhelmingly anytime AIDS is used in modern shows the underlying tone is negative or sarcastic. In nearly every joke made by a stand-up comedian the speaker uses AIDS, "I got an AIDS test," "how many of you are AIDS positive," "Oh no, my AIDS blood." When the topic is mentioned in satire or in a comedy show the "full blown AIDS" appears time and time again.

AIDS is not only used for humor, however; the choice of AIDS over HIV in a show was also made whenever the theme of punishment was also presented. For example, while discussing the need for testing Toni from *Girlfriends* uses HIV, "Can you believe Tod asked me to get an HIV test," but when addressing her guilt and fear the language shifts, "Maya, I'm telling you. Getting the AIDS will be my punishment." Nearly every show aired after 1995 used the term AIDS when making a point about the negative aspects of behavior.

When the goal of the show is providing facts, decreasing stigma, or encouraging behavior change, HIV is the language used. When characters are upset about their status and a family member, friend, or medical provider is attempting to calm the situation, again HIV is used. Take, for instance, in the 2008 episode of *Private Practice* (S2 E1), Dr. Freedman, Paul Adelstein, had just informed his teenage patient that he has HIV, "What am I going to tell people? Sorry I forgot I have AIDS?" to which Dr. Freedman quickly replies, "You don't have AIDS. OK, HIV. HIV, you take care of yourself you are going to live a long healthy life." In the conversation the teen is focused on the fear and perceived stigma he knows is attached to the virus, thus his use of AIDS. His doctor, however, understands that with medication and support the teen will be ok.

Overall most of the mentions of HIV were framed with information, offering a softening of the topic. The language sounded natural to the dialogue. While AIDS served as a means of jabbing the viewer, there is a harshness and edge to it's use. Never was a modern conversation about AIDS done without a deeper, and dominantly negative, connotation. Though a simple three letters, the use of HIV vs. AIDS illustrates the multiple levels of meaning this virus still carries with it.

NONVERBAL REACTIONS TO HIV

The final theme found across genres and time is the power of nonverbal communication. Words such as "you will be ok" and "HIV is no big deal" might be easy to say today, but reactions expressed through distancing and the awkward avoidance of touch speak volumes. Before people understood how HIV was transmitted fears of doorknobs, toilet seats, and sharing utensils were common. Upon hearing the words "I have HIV" the general reaction of anyone who does not understand the virus is likely to be seen taking a step back. Even if not a full step this physical pulling away is a clear signal of fear. Thus, the early days of the virus bred a fear of any form of touching. Yet, human touch is a vital component of existence. Knowing people are afraid to touch you, or even stand close, can therefore be one of the most isolating and stigmatizing experiences anyone can have.

Throughout the shows these nonverbal cues are shown repeatedly. Upon hearing a character is HIV-positive, 42 characters took a full step back, while an additional 32 leaned slightly back, all of whom also shifted their face to one of concern. One of the more blatant examples of physical reaction and fear is when Reesie (*Girlfriends* S3 E19) accidentally cuts herself while helping prepare dinner. Instantly, faces of horror with wide eyes and tight lips, each of the women not only back up but Maya and Toni quickly move to the other side of a counter. Acknowledging the fear, and also offering a moment of humor, Reesie explains what they need to do, "Guys its ok. I just get a trash can. We toss the veggies, toss the cutting board, and torch the whole kitchen. (pause) I am just kidding." Still in shock she continues, "Come on, guys, I feel awkward enough as it is." After still no movement from any of the friends, "Well can someone at least get me a Band-aid?" Finally, the women break from their trances and move in to offer help. Fear of positive blood is to be expected, however, fear of sharing a straw cuts a bit deeper.

During the episode of *21 Jump Street* (S2 E13), Hanson and Harley are in the cafeteria talking about living with HIV. Harley attempts to apologize to Hanson for being so much trouble,

> You know I wasn't always such a horse's ass. But dead men don't make friends easily. Especially with kids who don't think they are ever going to die. I just wish they weren't so afraid to even touch me. Nobody touches me anymore, man. Not my dad, hardly even my mom. It's the worst part. (dramatic pause) {laughs} Hey, I think I'm going to give them a pair of rubber gloves for their anniversary.

Not knowing how to respond Hanson looks down and states, "I, uh, I forgot my milk." Again, trying to make friends Harley offers his own milk, including the straw he had taken a sip from. After looking directly at the straw Hanson pauses and says, "Um uh, I don't like chocolate." Lowering his eyes and voice Harley quietly says, "Well yeah, no one does."

This moment with the milk not only becomes the moment Harley remembers as he refuses to return to school, but it's one of the moments he shares with his mother. When Hanson goes to the house to find Harley, the mother explains she was asked not to tell where he would be. "You make him feel like a leper." When asked in what way, she simply replies, "Next time, drink the milk. It won't kill you." Hanson finally finds Harley, and after a disrupted suicide attempt Harley's only request of Hanson is to be held, "I don't want to die, man. Can you do me a favor? Just hold me, man." Offering a full embrace of the teen the scene fades out. In the remaining moments of the episode the topic of the milk is mentioned for a final time. Harley's mother calls Hanson to inform him of Harley's passing; choking back tears she tells him, "He wanted me to let you know, it's ok about the milk."

Fear of touch from friends, family, even strangers would have been somewhat understandable given the uncertainty surrounding the virus. However, a lack of touch from medical providers is another story in itself. Though a refusal to touch an HIV-positive patient was never observed in a medical show, a handful of characters mention the situation. For example, in the episode of *Designing Women* Charlene is shown at only one point grabbing Kendall's hand. Noticing how he pauses and looks at her hands clasping his she asks what's the matter, "Oh nothing, you just surprise me. Taking my hand. Some of the nurses at the hospital even refused to come into my room" (S2 E4).

Such simple movements tell viewers quite a bit about the real fear experienced. Momentary pauses, and hesitant faces, scream even when a voice is silent. There is no risk in touching or even kissing someone with HIV, but on television it appears the characters have to be reminded of this from time to time. The modern HIV narratives do offer some better examples, but when screaming out "I have AIDS" in a waterpark the lines of people were still quick to take two steps back.

SUMMARY

With fewer shows including HIV themes within their narratives, the potential for viewers to gain awareness and knowledge about HIV through the narratives becomes even more important to consider. With six in ten young adults reporting that what they learn about HIV originates from television and other mediums, scholars must consider the rhetoric used within such shows. By focusing on the fundamental constructs of a genre, many implications prove problematic for the continued use of HIV narratives for reaction, ratings, or dramatic effect.

Thematically, shows must be presented in a probable manner. Unlike the "mental hygiene" films of the 1950s and the after school specials of the 70s and 80s, the themes may be probable, but many seem to be lacking in terms of being realistic. Scholars consistently report that when a viewer is transported into a show the messages presented within the show are often found less threatening and have a greater impact on behavior (Murphy 2011).

Nevertheless, rhetorical analysis illustrates that unlike many of the Grimm tales where evil often won, today's stories are far more likely to include a happily-ever-after ending. Characters, such as Christian from *Nip/Tuck*, are frequently shown engaging in risky behaviors with multiple women. The young adults of *Grey's Anatomy* engage in unprotected sex with each other and random characters. Then crisis arises and someone from the past reemerges with the threat of HIV. The characters fear that they too will be punished for their misdeeds, yet in the end most will be spared. This happily ever after, however, is not the case for 40,000 Americans each year.

Finally, the way in which HIV is discussed by medical practitioners as being "no big deal" enforces the presumption that viewers need not worry about testing or even prevention. These perceptions may also be enforced by the way the friends of those testing for HIV in the show talk about the issue. Additionally, the language about HIV being normal, or "the newest diabetes," may imply that there is no need to have the government worry about such issues. Therefore, funding to find a cure or better testing is also not needed.

Comments from friends, such as "you don't have it" and "you'll be fine" may persuade a viewer that they too will be fine. If Samantha from *Sex and the City* is "fine" after her test, then viewers can believe that their behavior, possibly being not nearly as risky as hers, wouldn't warrant the need of testing. On the other hand, framing HIV as a punishment as seen in many of the narratives may only enhance viewers' fears of testing. Fearing that they will be perceived as sluts, homosexuals, or drug dealers, thus inhibiting viewers' willingness to get tested.

It is clear that when shows take a strategic approach in their inclusion of HIV information, working with outside organizations such as the Kaiser Family Foundation, mediated narratives can be effectively disseminated prevention messages. However, many of the shows analyzed were not working with an outside organization, and may not have considered the implications of including an HIV plotline. Nonetheless, by examining these narratives it becomes apparent that regardless of intent, many lessons could be learned from these shows. It is clear that HIV is resented in a variety of probable situations; thus, offering viewers multiple opportunities to connect with the narratives. The next question is, are the characters themselves varied enough to allow for identification and parasocial relationships to be formed? Addressing this question, part three provides a deeper examination of the characters involved in the HIV narratives, viewers own voices about these shows, and finally the voices of some of the writers, producers, and actors.

NOTE

1. A character who contrasts with another character (usually the protagonist) in order to highlight particular qualities of the other character. In some cases, a subplot can be used as a foil to the main plot.

3

AIDS: The Body, The People, The Perceptions

Chapter Seven

Characters and the "AIDS Body"

In order for any lesson to be taught, critical decisions must be made in terms of who will spread the message. It is not just the situation that must be perceived as realistic by the audience but the characters themselves must also be engaging and relatable. It is the characters that bridge the audience to the lessons. Speaking to this directly, Kenneth Burke argues that often for persuasion to occur identification must also take place. Viewers are likely to be persuaded if they feel they share similar interests with a character. Therefore, if the goal is to teach the audience about their risk for HIV, the characters must be presented in a manner that encourages such identification. If this identification does not occur, Burke warns that distancing and division is likely. Thus, the potential for persuasion or education may be lost, when the audience is unable to connect with the character.

Burke is not alone in connecting identification with a character to persuasion and behavior change. Given the sensitive nature of talking about sexual health, communication scholars (Moyer-Gusé, Chung, & Jain 2011) argue that it is possible that mediated narratives are the only means of modeling such conversations. Providing characters for viewers to connect with allows them to observe and learn about the topic without feeling concerned they will say the wrong thing, or fear the personal consequences. For this connection to occur the viewers need to see themselves on the screen, including gender, race, age, social status, sexual orientation, and engagement of types of behavior.

BODIES AND BEHAVIOR

The behaviors observed, however, must also be carefully considered. HIV is transmitted a number of ways, but oftentimes shows make a point to emphasize stereotypes. One of the most explicit cases was in an episode of *House, MD.* Known for only taking on the "big deal" and interesting cases, on *House, MD* it was encouraging to find an episode involving an HIV-positive patient. Unfortunately, although facts about HIV are integrated into the show, far more stereotypes and common misperceptions are perpetuated. For instance, the character used to introduce the topic is quickly identified as a partying, drug using, gay man: a "PNP boy, party and play, drugs and sex" (*House, MD* S2 E7) as he labels himself. Other misperceptions arise as the doctors sit in a meeting discussing the case. Cameron, the young female doctor working closest with the patient, begins asking her colleagues if they always use condoms:

> Dr. Foreman: Ahhh. . . . Yeah.
>
> Dr. House: Brothers on the down low got to.
>
> Dr. Foreman: I am just not ready for any Foreman juniors. Yet.
>
> Dr. Cameron: You? (Addressing Dr. House)
>
> Dr. House: Working girls are sticklers.

Here, three dominant stereotypes are presented. The first is that all African American men are on the "down low," referring to men who (discreetly) have sex with other men (also referred to as MSM). Although young African American MSMs are one of the largest populations to seroconvert, anyone engaging in unprotected sex is at risk.

The second stereotype involves the reference to prostitutes. Again, although this is a high-risk population, drawing attention to these groups only perpetuates the idea that if one does not fit into one of these categories then he/she might not need to use condoms. Finally, Dr. Foremen's comment that he uses condoms to ensure he does not create a "junior" suggests condoms are efficacious only in pregnancy prevention, which ignores STD or HIV prevention. Although these statements are simple, the combination coupled with the abstention from any promotion for engaging in safe sexual behaviors leaves the responsibility of making the health connections to the audience.

Beyond prevention messages, showing an HIV-positive character that the viewer can personally connect with can help defuse fear and stigma about the illness. Showing prevention, testing, and living with the virus as a normal part of life is in many ways the only means of rupturing the taboo nature of HIV. Thus, the remainder of this chapter explores the various characters used to discuss HIV and AIDS. Looking not only at the behaviors that brought HIV into the story, but also the bodies themselves.

The Evolution of the AIDS Body

By the time AIDS had been given an official name, and was discussed by the media, thousands worldwide had already died. Therefore, it is not surprising that in the 80s and early 90s almost every character shown with HIV or AIDS died either by the end of the episode or within a few episodes. In total, looking across years and genres, more than 20 characters were shown, or directly mentioned, passing away from the virus. Interestingly, the three children shown with HIV are spared from the reality of HIV during that time. The only exception to this, *21 Jump Street*. Although not a "kid," Harley Poolish was the only character in high school that, after nearly taking his own life, ultimately dies of pneumonia in the last scene of the episode.

Mirroring news coverage, shows also began shifting from expected death to the challenges of living with the virus. Thus far, 27 HIV-positive characters have been given screen time. Take, for example, Josie in *A Different World*. Not only does she face the same concerns and fears of public speaking as her fellow classmates but she also has to overcome the stigma of living with a virus people still don't understand. Once her story is told classmates comment they will need to move dorms. The same student refuses to allow her to take a food order for fear of Josie touching the food. Not facing the same issues per se, other characters are shown facing discrimination from insurance companies and workplaces. By observing characters that look like and engage in the same activities as the viewer (going to class or work, dating, spending time with friends), it is easy to relate to the character. If show writers would have allowed Toni from *Girlfriends*, or Samantha from *Sex and the City*, or any character that an audience had already created a bond with, then when HIV is relived for that character, because a connection had already been made the audience member may be more likely to personally think about their own risk.

The late 90s and early 2000s shifted the focus by including more characters facing the possibility of contracting HIV. Within the majority of shows (including *Nip/Tuck*, *Grey's Anatomy*, even *Beverly Hills 90210*) it is only a secondary character who is depicted having the virus. The focus being placed on the central characters who now face the "punishment" for their past behaviors. Thus, for many, their whole world stops as they begin to fear the test, fear the judgment of those around them, and finally fear the results. Luckily for nearly all white, heterosexual, and non-drug-using characters the test will be negative. Resulting in more and more characters being saved from the consequences of their actions.

The lack of consequences become blatant when examining the times characters were tested in the show. As time and research progressed HIV-positive characters slowly became less of the focus, and testing and prevention messages spiked. In total, 24 characters have either been shown, or implied, that testing for HIV had occurred; 12 of which took place after 1998. Of those tested, 13 were gay, 12 straight, one was an intravenous drug user, and one was exposed to HIV-infected blood. When the results came in, only seven would come back positive. Five of the seven would be either gay or characters whom had shared a needle. Since 2003, only two additional characters have tested positive, both of whom were gay.

Unlike *Sex and the City*, where the central theme of the show is sex, shows such as *Designing Women*, *Girlfriends*, *The Parkers*, and *A Different World* are less likely to be thought of as a setting for HIV narratives. Consequently, a show such as the smash hit *Will and Grace*, whose cast is comprised of 50 percent gay characters, all whom frequently talk opening about a variety of other issued including homophobia, accepting a gay son, even adopting a gay horse, should be a prime location for an HIV narrative. Unfortunately, of the show's eight seasons, not a single episode took on the challenge.

In an interview with *POZ* magazine writers of the show spoke to the absence of the topic, "We talked about it from the beginning, But this was the first time there was going to be a gay male lead on TV. We wanted him to be healthy and happy." It should be noted that *Will and Grace* did briefly mentioned HIV once, when Grace went in for a doctor's appointment. However, the mention never developed into anything more. The writer states, "In real life, they would have been around HIV for 20 years, but we decided that Will and Grace should live in a fantasy world," says Poust. The opportunity was missed for *Will and Grace*, however, when compared to how other shows have chosen to incorporate the topic of HIV, the choice of living in a fantasy world might be providing the better option.

Today, although rarely seen, HIV-positive characters appear to live normal lives. In fact an HIV-positive character has not been shown dying of the virus since the graceful exit of Vic in season four of *Queer as Folk* in 2004. When an HIV-positive character is introduced, it is a means of a larger goal. This goal being to explain or advance a medical or dramatic situation. Or, as is the case with comedies, a joke is needed as a means of extra edge. One show, however, provides an HIV-positive character, without any of the stereotypical storylines. In the show *Looking*, Eddie Bear's character does not provide the typical testing story. He simply is HIV positive, it's part of who he is but not the only part. Thus, the show provides the furthest evolved narratives on television.

THE EMBODIMENT OF AIDS

One of the struggles early on in the HIV epidemic was a lack of personal connection to the virus. It wasn't until Magic Johnson and Ryan White became public that people and the media really took notice. Finally, the media had a "face" for editors to post on newspapers, magazine covers, and television screens. With the earliest case of HIV and AIDS primarily being found within drug use and gay populations the immediate danger was that audiences would assume that these were the only populations at risk. Therefore, writers and casting directors had to make careful choices in the characters that would embody HIV and AIDS in the shows. Considering who is speaking for HIV, by living or dying from the illness, shapes viewers perceptions as they often create the first memory of "meeting" someone with the illness. Looking across the decades three categories of embodiment were found; the sick, the victims, and the villains.

The Sick. Echoing the early days of the virus, shows dominantly shaped perceptions by emphasizing the "illness" aspects of HIV. In fact, the only two characters portrayed as having the illness were shown gaunt and sick. In the most extensive case, the character on *House* was also suffering from additional illness. Even with many of the characters in the late 80s and early 90s, most the HIV-positive characters appeared healthy looking. When they became sick, and ultimately passed away, on the show they were rarely observed. Instead the death is hidden either by fading to the funeral scene or a conversation is had about their death. However, many of the characters are shown visibly upset by their conditions: for instance, the majority of the characters' medical issues such as seeking an abortion, being the only possible donor match for a sibling, or trying to understand some other "mystery illnesses." Yet sickness was not the only way in which HIV could be embodied by a character. Others were shown dealing with everyday issues such as helping friends understand the illness and how to adapt to having a friend with HIV. Other depictions included the typical situation of having to disclose to previous partners the need for testing, as well as the less common issue of a teen finding out for the first time that he has HIV or characters having to go to court to help prosecute someone for knowingly infecting others with HIV.

The Victims. Across nearly all the dramatic representations of HIV narratives characters are portrayed as either the victim or villain. According to Burke, guilt, purification, and redemption are required elements for maintaining social order. Seeing dramas as a means of teaching moral lessons, the goal became clear that in order to perpetuate societal expectations examples of those who rejected the hierarchy or order would need to be punished. As mentioned previously this level of guilt is commonly remedied through conversations and actions taken within the time span of one episode. However, for the characters already shown living with the virus the victims often become those who contract HIV not because of their own actions, but because of the actions of others. For example, within the show *Girlfriends* Reesie, the young African American woman, contracted HIV, which had progressed to

AIDS, from her husband. Not wanting to be labeled as gay, Reesie's husband refused to use a condom when engaging in sexual activity with other men; subsequently passing the virus to his wife Reesie.

Similar to Reesie, the majority of other women shown having contracted HIV are portrayed as victims of either misplaced trust in their partners or outright targeting. More than 15 female characters were passed HIV by boyfriends or partners they stated they trusted and loved. Only a handful of female characters were framed as being engaged with multiple partners, and even fewer contracted HIV from the use of drugs. Men on the other hand were rarely ever painted as the victim. The exception to the rule being any male teen or child. In each case where a child was HIV-positive, each show was quick to explain that the cause was from either blood transfusion, or passed down from the mother. However, transmission from the mother only occurred once.

For those portrayed as characters living with HIV, statements such as "I have it," "this disease," and "I have AIDS" became telling signs of how the character felt about their condition as well as how the viewers might frame the illness within their own minds. Characters employing statements of distance, such as "I have it," or "this disease" make it apparent that HIV is not, and was not, something they sought to experience. As a result, this failure to name HIV as a disease may mark for the viewer that it is shameful and something worthy of being feared. A few of the characters speak frankly about the struggle this illness has created; however, little beyond mentioning these struggles is ever shown to the audience.

What makes Reesie (*Girlfriends*) different from all the other victims of HIV is the use of the phrase "my AIDS." Such a phrase indicates that this illness is something she has learned to accept. Seeing her HIV as something that belongs to her rather than the disease acting on her provides a sense of agency instead of the shameful victimhood implied by labeling HIV as "it" or "the disease." It is now a part of who she is; while it is not everything, it is a part of her.

The Villains. In juxtaposition to the victims are the villains of HIV. In some cases villains are shown using HIV as a weapon (i.e., *CSI:NY*, *Law and Order: SVU*). Consistently played by a male character, this type of villain purposely seeks out to infect as many others as possible. Feeling as if they have been wronged by some outside force these men seek out both men and women whom they can infect. In four different shows characters state directly that what has happened to them was not fair, claiming to be victims themselves, however, as a means of coping they lash out to punish others for engaging in risky behaviors, "They are getting what they deserve" (*Law and Order: SVU*).

Then again not all villains were male. Women were also found to be cast in a similar role. Unlike the previous category these women have only potentially given their "disease" to the central character. In each case this villain is an ex-partner who has returned to destroy the now happy life. Portrayed as being hyper sexual, a prostitute, liar, or drug user each of the female villains is beyond saving, and will therefore only have one or two episodes to tell their tale. In contrast to the male villains these characters were also less likely to be accused of spreading the virus on purpose. Not a single example could be found where HIV was used by a female character as a weapon.

Finally, villains were also depicted by companies or policies directly targeting people living with HIV. These villains included insurance companies refusing to cover medication, employers finding other candidates when sexual orientation is implied, even landlords refusing to house characters living with HIV. In each instance, the shows mirrored real-life situations people living with HIV were, and still are, facing. It is in these situations that the larger lessons learned provide the valuable insight into the daily life and struggle of people living with HIV. With medications HIV is treatable, but with the overwhelming stigma and discrimination hiding in the shadows of policy and red tape it's almost impossible to defeat these types of monsters.

MISSING REPRESENTATIONS

Although a diverse cast of characters is found across the decades and genres, significant holes existed. Foremost is the lack of homosexual African American men and Latinos, regardless of sexual orientation. Latino men may be modeled in telenovelas, however, these were not included in the present analysis. The absence of these populations not only inaccurately portrays the issue, but also neglects to offer a character for viewers to connection to while modeling how these populations could approach topics of HIV. According to the CDC (2014), among men who had been diagnosed with HIV or AIDS who had become infected through male-to-male sexual contact, 56 percent were black/African American, 65 percent were Hispanic/Latino, and 79 percent were white. Among women diagnosed with HIV or AIDS who had become infected through heterosexual contact, 78 percent were black/African American, 75 percent were Hispanic/Latina, and 68 percent were white (CDC, 2014). Based on the conventions represented within television shows, the normalcy of talking about testing is not as common for African American and Latino men (both straight or gay) as it is for their white counterparts. With these populations left out of the conversation internalized discrimination, stigmatization, and fear are perpetuated. By not including their story, viewers lack the ability to observe that HIV impacts everyone, regardless of race, age, and sexual orientation.

Also missing from the discussion of HIV in television are multiple representations of college-aged adults. In the 80s, *A Different World* provided both college-aged and African American characters. In the late 90s, *Beverly Hills, 90210* served as a model starting off with the characters shown in high school and then in college, where the HIV episode took place. It was not until 2015 that another college-aged character, Oliver (Conrad Ricamora) in *How to get away with Murder*, is shown. As a result, HIV would appear to only rarely impact college settings.

Although HIV is no longer a death sentence the numbers of new infections have continued to increase. Unfortunately, however, if the discussion of HIV in television was any indication, it would see HIV is in fact no big deal. As it would seem that the need to talk about HIV in shows is no longer a topic worth discussing. In total, since 2006, only 11 episodes have included either HIV-positive characters or a discussion of risk for HIV. With such few voices speaking out about the risks for HIV it is no wonder why young people feel it's no longer an issue.

SUMMARY

To increase the likelihood of connection between viewers and characters, each character should be both relatable and believable to the viewers. When examining the characters portrayed within the shows discussing HIV, the character becomes increasingly important given the stigma and numerous stereotypes already attached to those living with HIV. In the beginning of the epidemic many shows portrayed HIV patients as being white homosexual males often shown as gaunt, sickly, and covered in lesions. This representation is problematic given that anyone can become infected with HIV. If a viewer is only able to observe the worst and extreme cases of HIV and AIDS it is likely they will assume the symptoms of the illness would be obvious, and testing would not be needed.

If television shows were to represent HIV using a variety of backgrounds and characteristics, viewers may be better able to see how HIV could affect them. Many stereotypes pervade portrayals of AIDS-positive characters: having used intravenous drugs, homosexuals, and a few who have had numerous partners or met people online for anonymous sex. Fortunately, a wide variety of bodies were used across the shows including men, women, heterosexuals, homosexuals, Caucasians, African Americans, young people, and people in their sixties. Further, a few specific characters have helped break down the misconception of who is a risk. *Grey's Anatomy*, *Private Practice*, and *Without a Trace* included young Caucasian heterosexual women, *Law and Order* as well as *Private Practice* also focused attention on young heterosexuals. This lack of range in terms of backgrounds, races, and experiences limit the possibility for others to identify with the character while also learning that HIV is something that affects only certain groups. Thus, a great deal more is needed in terms of the embodiment of HIV if stigma and misperceptions are ever going to be eliminated.

Chapter Eight

Negative in Life, Positive on Screen

Without talking directly to the writers, producers, and actors involved in mediated HIV narratives it is impossible to know what an episode intended to achieve. Luckily, when HIV narratives are presented on television the press often takes notice. As a result, interviews with actors, writers, even directors and producers of these shows provide a glimpse behind the screen, and illuminate the choices made in many of the shows. Examining the conversation surrounding portrayals of HIV on television, and a personal discussion with an actor who has played a few HIV-positive roles on stage and screen, this chapter provides a second lens of the perception of HIV on television.

WHY HIV ON TELEVISION?

Even with countless news reports covering AIDS during the 80s talking about any topic related to sex in a television show was considered taboo. Layering on the almost certain death that accompanied AIDS early on, and a population already experiencing stigma, taking on the issue of AIDS in a television show was considered a risky move. Therefore, *why* HIV was a repeated question throughout countless interviews with writers and producers of the shows where an HIV narrative was included.

Taking note of how sensitive topics such as uterine cancer, the importance of PAP smears, and abortion had been delicately handled in early episodes of *Guiding Light*, the producers of *General Hospital* felt they had an important role to play when it came to educating audiences about AIDS. In an interview with *Entertainment Weekly*, executive producer Wendy Riche states, "We were going to show the audience that knowledge [about AIDS] is power." The inclusion of not one but two characters with AIDS quickly caught the attention of the media and began to receive high praise, "*General Hospital* producers' timely message was one of compassion for victims of the AIDS epidemic and raised awareness that anyone could contract the virus not just homosexuals and drug addicts." Other interviews with the show's writers indicated some obvious trepidation, but ultimately writers noted seeing a gross amount of misunderstanding about the virus, and felt they could help. Taking a targeted approach of showing that anyone could get AIDS, Michael Sutton (the actor who played the first HIV-positive character on the show, Stone Cates) and the cast of *General Hospital* achieved their goal of raising awareness, and provided a spark that inspired many subsequent shows not only in the world of soap operas, but also on primetime.

General Hospital, however, was not the first show to take on the topic; years before in another hospital a doctor discovered he had contracted the virus. Tom Fontana, a producer of *St. Elsewhere*, explains that the inclusion of AIDS as a topic was a means of showing audiences the consequences of the sexual freedom people had grown accustom to. Fontana tells the *Chicago Tribune*, "We wanted to look at sexual freedom and an entire generation's attitude toward free love. For the last 15 years or so, we were told that free love was okay, but now it's catching up with us. And most of the people who watch our show probably are those who have been out there for 15 years making love with various partners." Rupturing the ideology of free love not only offered a window into the consequences of sexual behavior but it also brought the topic of sexual health as a whole into view.

Dissecting Hollywood's struggle to talk about HIV, CNN reporter Jeanne Bonner interviewed David Caplan, a celebrity journalist and former editor at *People* magazine. In the interview Caplan is quoted discussing that the AIDS crisis as a "taboo" topic, making it a challenging topic for popular culture to address. Given the taboo surrounding any unknown and stigmatizing issue, such as HIV, shows often had to use "unusual approaches." Caplan states, "It [talking about AIDS] was always done from afar and often involving a heterosexual character, which was good because it was trying to normalize it." Caplan continues, "But it was also questionable in terms of how realistic it was. It was a disease that was ravaging the gay community." Offering an example Caplan takes note of the straight white women of *Golden Girls*, "I like it, I get it, but it's not realistic." The balance of normalizing AIDS while also being realistic continues to challenge writers and producers to date.

A more modern struggle of portraying HIV in a realistic manner was *Queer as Folk*. The show provided an HIV-positive main character in the second season. However, some of the viewers felt even this representation was inaccurate. In an article for *HIVplus* magazine Benjamin Ryan provides a wealth of opinion on the show as well as "Hollywood's version of HIV" in general. In his interview with Martin Hollick, a man who has lived with HIV for 17 years, Ryan asks about the realness of *Queer as Folk*. "No one on earth looks as good as Ben" (the character in the show). "And certainly no one I know with HIV looks like that. He was on his deathbed at the hospital, and he looked better than I do after a week at the spa. OK, it's TV no sunken cheeks." Ben's appearances began in 2004, a time that had already forgotten the death sentence HIV once was. To Hollick's point, the use of the "sick" HIV body, highlighted by a skinny build and sunken cheeks, has not been seen on television since the late 90s.

Although Ben's character might not have been completely realistic the show is praised for approaching HIV boldly and from a variety of angles including the reality of taking HIV medications. Creators of *Queer as Folk*, Ron Cowen and Daniel Lipman, state, "there seems to be a lot of irresponsible behavior going on, and a lot of misinformation regarding the medications." For instance, one of the characters, Vic, was used to address the reality that commonly people living with HIV die not because of the virus, but due to the side effects of the medications. For both Cowen and Lipman accurate information about the medications and life with HIV was something desperately needed on television. In part, this need stemmed from the increased numbers of people taking the medications. With more people on medications, thus living longer with this virus, the need to show other aspects of life with HIV has also inspired shows to weave in longer threads of HIV.

The need for medical information also grew from the overall lack of accurate portrayals of HIV risk. From HIV vigilantes to the epidemic of young straight people who contract HIV through a blood transfusion, the general method of normalizing HIV for anyone who wasn't gay was to include a character who contracts the virus from an outside source. Even worse, the majority of HIV-positive characters shown on television in the 80s were straight white women.

Women who had been cheated on by a husband, fooled by a charming man, or attacked. Only in the show *Nip/Tuck* was a woman with HIV framed as "deserving" HIV. In other words, shown both directly and indirectly engaging in behaviors related with risk.

Author of the book *The Prime-Time Closet*, Stephen Tropiano, argues that one of the primary reasons realistic depictions of HIV-positive people are difficult to find is because the creators are attempting to cast as wide of a net as possible. It is understood that viewership is broad, thus networks seek to use the broadest brush as possible, in hopes of not offending potential viewers. Overwhelmingly, the majority of shows focus on white viewers. Thus, networks including ABC, NBC, and CBS commonly refrain from including African Americans, Latinos, Asians, and gay characters as a whole. In Tropiano's book he states, "It really comes down to selling advertising time and ratings, and as a result of that, everything is pretty mainstream." Based on this logic, Tropiano further explains, "You don't see [HIV-positive people] because there's no money in it and because they [networks] want to stay as far away from controversy as they can." Tropiano is not wrong in pointing out that including HIV in a storyline often comes with controversy.

Not afraid of offending viewers, or of controversy, Jackie Marcus Schaffer and Jeff Schaffer, creators of the show *The League*, were interviewed by June Thomas, managing editor of *Slate*, a daily web magazine. Finding the character "douchey" Thomas thought it was incredibly odd to see the other characters of the show becoming jealous of his "full blown AIDS" status. As a result, Thomas contacted the show creators to understand the divisions behind the character. Jackie explains, "I was literally making a chopped salad for dinner as our baby is asleep, and I said, 'Let me just throw something at you: Ted has AIDS.' Because what is more insane that a bunch of guys trying to figure out if somehow the AIDS has made him more successful and more focused." As simple as that the character's status was decided, and the topic was woven into the episode. Questioning the appropriateness of this choice Thomas asks the duo, "So there are no sacred cows in *The League*'s comedy?" Taking the question Jeff states, "I do think that a lot of shows wouldn't touch this, and we're very happy to. We're not looking to shock, we're just looking for what's funny, but this is a real thing that you don't see a lot of stories about." Ted's character, luckily, is short lived and soon he becomes far too busy for the friends and the show moves on without him. Similar to many comedy shows the topic of HIV and AIDS is tossed in for a joke and then simply left without much of a repercussion. The same, however, cannot be said for all shows.

HIV AND THE DEMISE OF SHOWS THAT INCLUDE IT

Days after Dr. Caldwell, of *St. Elsewhere*, was told he had AIDS, Steve Daley of the *Chicago Tribune* had something to say. In his article titled *St. Elsewhere Contracts A Problem With AIDS*, Daley sharply criticizes the show and the "ghoulish fascination with AIDS that has swept through prime-time network programing." Not only critiquing *St. Elsewhere* Daley also poignantly addresses the inclusion of AIDS in the shows such as *Hotel* and *Mr. Belvedere* finding the stories "slapped together around AIDS for Friday night viewing." Yet, according to Daley, "The risks are far greater for *St. Elsewhere*, 'a decent program with an audience consisting of people who know their ZIP codes from their area codes. When not much is demanded (e.g., "Hotel"), not much is expected. A choice like the one being made in Wednesday`s episode, where Caldwell learns that he has apparently contracted the illness through contact with a female prostitute, could undo almost four years of good will with a devoted but critical audience.'" Daley was, however, not alone in questioning the impact the AIDS storyline would have on viewers.

When another largely successful show, *Life Goes On*, wrote in an HIV-positive diagnosis for Jesse (Chad Lowe) the ultimate health of the show was brought into question. Greg Dawson, writer for the *Orlando Sentinel*, praises the show as being "the only series dealing with the disease in a realistic manner," however, based on an interview with Bob Iger, an executive of ABC, the chances of the show being renewed were looking "comparatively slim." In fact, the show would indeed not see another season. While HIV does take Jesse's life in the end, there is no evidence of the HIV storyline also being the killer of the show.

Though shows such as *Life Goes On*, *Designing Women*, and *ER* received praise for the handling of HIV in the storyline many others were closely dissected, and found to be overwhelmingly missing the mark. Choosing to weave in an HIV-positive character in it's last season, in ABC's *Brothers and Sisters*, Uncle Saul's testing experience was found to be missing multiple opportunities to portray reality. At the time, 2011, Saul was the only HIV-positive character in a regular or recurring role on television in the United States. That said, while having a character wait until the next day for results provided dramatic tension, the reality is modern HIV tests typically only take twenty minutes. Not to mention the legal ramifications for giving results over the phone. It is Sarah Audelo, Senior Manager of *Advocate for Youth* who specifically calls into question this phone call. Recounting the scene, Audelo calls out the scene as fail for not only the way in which Saul reacts to the results, he smiles and lies to his family, but also the fact that the whole conversation lasts less than a minute. "When someone tests positive, we want to get them into care immediately. Whether it's explaining what exactly it means to be HIV positive, providing counseling, answering questions, discussing options, learning about resources for those who are HIV positive . . . it's a whole package of services that need to happen so we don't lose people who quite honestly could be feeling overwhelmed with what many still think is a death sentence. Hence the ten second phone call, FAIL." Failing even more, according to the Buzzfeed News reporter Louis Peitzman is *How to Get Away With Murder* (*HTGAWM*).

Calling out the show for it's "after-school-special" feel Peitzman critiques not only the choice of including HIV in the storyline, but also the manner through which it is handled.

> On the one hand, it's refreshing to see a television series once again tackling the subject of HIV, which has all but disappeared from the TV landscape. (Until Thursday night's *HTGAWM* finale, Eddie, played by Daniel Franzese, on HBO's *Looking* was the only HIV-positive character on a current series.) But on the other, the show's approach to HIV was an embarrassing representation of *HTGAWM*'s muddled queer politics: Connor continues to alternate between a progressive representation of a sexually liberated gay man and a

> caricature who's defined solely by his bedroom activities and slut-shamed for his promiscuity.

Offering ABC some praise for the unapologetic and sexually liberated character Connor, played by Jack Falahee, Peitzman notes "there's never been a character like Connor on network television before. His sexual escapades rival those of Brian (Gale Harold) on Showtime's *Queer as Folk*, and he's wholly unapologetic about his random hookups. Which is a beautiful thing. The ABC series deserves plenty of credit for taking things as far as it has." That said, Peitzman finds the storyline "pedantic and condescending" explaining that, "When Connor went in for his HIV test, he was lectured on his safe sex practices. It was disappointing to see that a character presented as sexually uninhibited had no idea he could contract HIV from topping, and that he seemed unclear as to why he and Oliver both had to get tested before they could resume sexual contact." To this point Peitzman is not alone. Other reviewers of the show also shared the opinion that *HTGAWM* had digressed back decades to where people didn't know unprotected sex could have serious repercussions. However, the primary fault Peitzman appears to find is that it is not Connor, fitting of the stereotype, that contracts HIV. Discussing the irony of the "clean-cut, sexually responsible" Oliver finding out he's HIV positive Peitzman states, it

> felt like another lesson to be learned: *Anyone can contract HIV!* It's territory that was covered by any number of TV series throughout the '80s and '90s. It's quite the paradox that *How to Get Away With Murder*, which has been painted as a forward-thinking series for its inclusion of Connor as well as its diverse cast, is presenting the same ideas that were on television three decades earlier.

In the end Peitzman is accurate, fewer characters are shown talking about, let alone living with, HIV. Those that do are rarely given the opportunity to truly portray the reality of the illness in today's society.

Essentially, it appears that portraying HIV accurately is not always the goal of the writers and producers. For some the motivation behind the inclusion of HIV was with the goal of raising awareness and educating audiences, for others HIV is simply a means of getting the laugh or creating dramatic effect. Thankfully, the same motivation does not seem to be the case for the actors playing the role.

PERCEPTIONS OF THE ACTORS

Even more common than interviewing a writer about the use of HIV in a storyline, are interviews with the actors playing the characters. While working with AIDS Watch 2016 in Washington, DC, a once in a lifetime opportunity was given to interview Daniel Franzese from HBO's show *Looking*. Playing the incomparable character Eddie (known as "Bear"), Franzese brings a powerful voice to the screen, finally providing for viewers a realistic portrayal of HIV on television. Combining my own interview with Franzese and published interviews, the following offers the perspective of the men and women who have played an HIV-positive character.

Why These Characters?

Knowing how stigmatizing HIV is, a viewer may wonder why any actor would take on such a role. For Michael Sutton, the first actor to play an HIV-positive character on a soap opera, the feelings surrounding the opportunity were mixed,

> When I was acting I knew I needed to portray it correctly, and to have the delicacy to do that. But, I did not want to be the poster boy for AIDS foundations and things like that, because in a way, I did not want to be pigeonholed, and wanted my work to stand on its own. And, not necessarily go on and fight for a cause, and not be able to be separated from the two for an acting career. It was selfishly just for the career.

For Gloria Reuben, the actress who played Jeanie Boulet on *ER* the idea of playing an HIV-positive character was met with feelings of trepidation. However, having known someone with the virus helped her see that the story needed to be told. During a panel discussion with The Elizabeth Taylor AIDS Foundation (ETAF) Reuben was joined by fellow ambassador/actor Daniel Franzese (*Looking*), writer/producer Neal Baer (*ER*, *Law & Order: SVU*) and ETAF's Managing Director Joel Goldman. Meeting to discuss HIV-positive characters on television a *Variety* magazine reporter was able to gather and share these iconic viewpoints. Ruban recounts, "I had the feeling, rightfully so, that this was going to be tough for a long time because still, it's my face out there on this." To which she was correct, her face remained the face of HIV for years after the show ended. In fact Reuben's character would be the only main HIV-positive character in a show until Robert Gant's character, Ben, entered the screen on *Queer as Folk* in 2002.

Reuben was not the only actor to take on an HIV positive role because of having personal connection to the virus. Franzese also explained that while he had known a few people with the virus it wasn't until talking about the character for *Looking* had overlapped a personal friend's recent diagnosis that he felt the need to get involved in HIV advocacy. For both Franzese and Reuben these characters were not simply another character they would play, but an opportunity to get involved in something bigger than themselves.

Similarly, Anthony Azizi, who played the HIV-positive Special Assistant to the President, Vince Taylor, on ABC's show *Commander in Chief*, wanted to stand for something. In an interview with *POZ* magazine he states, "My family is Middle Eastern, and that culture is very nervous about HIV, because to them it means "gay" and gay is a real hot button. I'm from Iran, raised in New York and Philadelphia, and being from that heritage, I understand the stigma that's attached to HIV. But in order to accept someone with HIV, you have to accept them for being human. We're all brothers and sisters—we're all truly connected—and we have to care." Not only was Azizi the first and only Iranian actor to portray an HIV-positive character on television, this is the closest HIV has ever been to the White House in terms of a fictional show. Speaking to this directly Dee Johnson, executive producer (and occasional co-writer) of the show, "We're all aware that [HIV has] fallen off the radar in perception but not in reality. So why not put a person with that situation right into the biggest, most powerful place on earth?"

Unlike many of the other actors who walked into a show knowing the status of a character, Conrad Ricamora, a fellow actor, told Oliver on *How to Get Away with Murder*, that he would be testing positive. Ricamora tells *Plus Magazine*'s Daniel Reynolds, about those first moments. "I just stood there, stunned, staring off into space . . . like I had just found out a real person tested positive, and going through all the grief and denial." Once the news of his character's status had time to sink in he recalls, "I remember growing up in the '90s, it was such a big educational topic. . . . [But] in the last couple of years, it's slid out of the consciousness of mainstream America. It's a huge honor to be able to bring this back into the consciousness."

Although playing Oliver was an honor for Ricamora it seemed the fans were not so accepting. He shares, "Some people are really, really heartbroken and sad. People come up to me and tell me all the time, 'Oh! I cried so much when I found out!' Just a lot of sad people, because, I guess, everybody loves Oliver." Hearing directly from fans as well, Franzese shared, "I have gotten a lot of feedback from people who have seen Eddie on *Looking.* They have told me that it gives them hope to be able to see the same things they face in their own relationships happening in the show." It is the ability to show viewers people they can identify with that Franzese argues is key for advancing the HIV narrative. "Being able to see yourself on the screen helps you feel valid and accepted. That is really important."

More from Daniel Franzese

Not limited by what has been edited and published I had the unique opportunity to ask Franzese to share his experiences playing Eddie as well as the role he felt media could play in preventing the continued spread of HIV. The following interview speaks not only of Franzese's clear understanding of how impactful media can be, but also his call for what media needs to be doing.

What are your thoughts on the way HIV has been discussed in popular culture?

> Early on the message was on understanding and the facts of HIV, and how people can protect themselves. But where we are now I feel that with 1.2 people living with the virus in the US and only 3 characters telling that story on television, we are not doing enough.

What characters (or shows), in television, do you feel have done an effective job talking about HIV?

> We have had a lot of great shows that have talked about what HIV was like in the past, but we are seriously lacking what it's like now and the future. It's only a small mention in some shows, such as the brief mention on *Transparent*, and like a C line story in *How to Get Away with Murder*. But being on *Looking*, we are the first show to talk about PReP. We are also showing a couple and the real problems that can arise. The story of Eddie is in many ways revolutionary with how brave he is. His focus is not on his HIV status, but he is shown living in spite of it.

What do you hope people will learn from watching Eddie?

> For Eddie HIV is just a part of his life. So I hope for others who are positive this can be true as well. That everyone has the right to love and be loved like everyone else.

How have you prepared for this role?

> I was going through the beginning stages of a close friend finding out he was positive. When I was offered the character I was told his status would not be a big thing in the character's life. It would just be something that happened.

Do you think that was the right way to approach the topic?

> Yes, I don't think it needs to be big thing. This portrayal takes his story and shows how he turned his life around. For Eddie HIV was the catalyst for change. He once was a wild guy going out to clubs, but when he discovers he is positive he starts focus on helping others. He starts working in the shelter for homeless and trans folk. I really think this was a great way to shape the character.

How can we make this happen?

> Just keep talking about it. That's how people are now accepting Trans issues across multiple platforms because it's not a popular topic to discuss. The same needs to happen with HIV. It seems HIV has taken a backseat to those other

movements and they are all important, but I feel like we need as a community to bring that issue back to the forefront.

HIV used to be a really popular topic for the media to talk about; why do you think it's fallen off the radar?

People are living a lot longer now, so the fear is gone. So those stories are just not being told. But people don't realize how expensive it is to be HIV positive. They don't know how much these medications and treatments cost. I think it's something around $400,000 to treat HIV each year. That message is not getting out there. And I think there are some major pharmaceutical companies that don't want that message out there.

Do you think these characters can play a role in educating viewers?

Yes, it's very similar to the ways characters have educated audiences about LGBT populations in general. Someone might not know someone who has HIV, but by seeing their favorite characters, like seeing Oliver and Connor in *How to Get Away with Murder* getting tested, you are able to say "oh that's my friend." You feel the same emotions, and understand the issues that arise surrounding treatment and prevention when you see someone else go through it. TV can reach a lot of people and change a lot of minds faster than any wall can. I really feel that the more people are talking about HIV and AIDs the more people can learn. Popular culture has a huge role to play in getting us to talk. What needs happen is we need to see testing without it being a whole show about HIV. I would love to see a character on *The New Girl* go get tested for HIV. We need to see this happening all the time without it being a special episode. Just make it a routine thing.

In multiple interviews Franzese provides a variety of ways HIV can be brought to the attention of viewers. Including the continuation of characters like Oliver on popular shows such as *How to Get Away with Murder*. Research suggests that viewers can learn from watching the characters they like, and as an actor Franzese himself is hoping this connection is being made. However, without directly asking viewers it's impossible to know. Providing the final lens of perception, chapter nine presents the findings of two studies involving interviews with young viewers.

Chapter Nine

"Those People Are at Risk"

Media's ability to influence viewer perceptions of HIV remains crucial in the prevention of HIV, given that television offers many viewers their only exposure to HIV and sexual health education (Brown, Steele, & Walsh-Childers 2001). In order to understand if the HIV narratives presented on television were in fact shaping perceptions of young adults an online survey was sent out and one-on-one interviews were scheduled. Over six hundred online surveys were collected, with questions focusing on where participants learn about HIV, if/which of the narratives discussed in the previous chapters had been seen, as well as a fifty-item true/false quiz testing knowledge of HIV. Delving further an additional 115 interviews, with college students of three universities, have been conducted. These interviews asked participants to reflect on what they recall seeing in the media about HIV, who they felt is at risk, and where their knowledge has come from.

Largely the quantitative portions of these studies indicated that college students do have a healthy understanding of what places a person at risk for HIV. They do not believe HIV can be contracted from a toilet or telephone. Nor do young people feel that being around others living with the virus will put themselves at risk. However, throughout the interview phase it became clear that college students do not have an accurate perception of risk when it comes to their own behaviors. Overall, participants felt the coverage of HIV has largely focused attention only on specific groups, and rarely (if ever) has that attention been on young adult populations. Providing insight into young adults' perceptions of HIV the following chapter highlights the young adult viewer's abilities to connect with, and learn from, HIV narratives presented on television.

PERCEPTIONS OF HIV

With research maintaining that young adult populations do not personally connect with HIV, the first research question asked what college students' perceptions are, in terms of risk for HIV. What was identified is that overwhelmingly participants felt HIV is not framed by the media as a problem in the United States, is a topic that is too taboo to be discussed, and that while certain groups are at risk college students do not consider their actions risky.

General Perceptions of Risk for HIV

The college students interviewed for this study shared an accurate understanding of what would put someone at risk for HIV. Therefore, it was not surprising that when asked to define risk for HIV, many participants focused on the transfer of fluids. For example Kayla stated, "Anyone who is sexually active. Anyone who is a drug user and shares needles. Anyone who gets any kind of blood. Or a mother who doesn't know and has a child."[1] Kathryn also focused on the fluid aspect of risk, "Any kind of fluid contact. Blood, semen, but not saliva." Going a bit further in depth, Heather noted, "Any types of bodily fluid that you would come into contact from another person. I know you can't get it from saliva but semen, vaginal fluids, blood, any contact or during other outbreaks of other STDs."

Many others found risk to be less technical, and felt risk for HIV was as simple as having unprotected sex, "Risk is anything unprotected. Not thinking before you act is a risk," Holly explained. Similarly, Heather indicated that one must also be smart about their behaviors, "I think you just have to be smart about what you are doing and who are you with." Although young adults' knowledge scores have been found to be consistently high, the theme of "needing to be smart" about HIV and particularly who you are with, remained a common theme when asked about what would put someone at risk for HIV. Conrad states, "I guess having a lack of knowledge and participating in activities with others who have it. I think they need to know the real ways of contracting it. As long as the person who has HIV and the person who does not are not together or have knowledge of how it can happen people should be all right." When asked who would be at risk for HIV, Conrad continued, "People without knowledge to a point. Like any other disease, it's easy to pick up if you don't know how to protect yourself." The issue is, however, that based on their knowledge scores college students are "smart" in terms of knowing about HIV and should know better. Yet many remain unable to put this knowledge into action.

Prevalence of HIV in the United States

Participants were each directly asked if they felt HIV was shown as a problem in the United States by the media. While a few did comment that it is a problem everywhere, most felt that, given the lack of discussion about HIV on television, that it may not be as big of a problem as in Africa. Anna notes, "We only want to know about ourselves. So we don't tend to care about other people. Unless it is a natural disaster that kills a ton of people. Like nobody here cares that 1 or 2 people are dying of HIV and AIDS every second in Africa." Heather also remarked that HIV is not seen as a problem in our society anymore. She finds that the focus "Has been directed to the third world countries, like Africa." Anna also explains, "It's not really an epidemic here anymore. Maybe just more for the partiers, there it is more likely."

This idea that HIV was once a problem in the United States was also mentioned by Mark who said, "I think years ago it was shown more as a problem than now." Resonating with the other participants, Ben reflects on his training in the military has taught soldiers that HIV is not a problem in the United States, "I remember in our military briefings, Africa is like 40% HIV positive by itself. It is going to kill their whole country. They have a problem. We have a lack of protection where it could become a problem." Similarly, others agreed that HIV is just not as big of a problem in the United States. Taylor explained, "I think it's a problem in low-income areas of the world because people are not able to receive the types of contraceptives that are needed to have safe sex, but that is not the case for the US."

These comments as well as others offer support to Tufte's (2005) argument that for many young adults, the perception is that HIV is only taking place in forgotten or unfamiliar worlds. If their perception is that HIV is not impacting their world, then it seems logical they would not be personally concerned they are at risk.

Perceptions of Who Is at Risk for HIV

In general, participants had two categories for who would be at risk for HIV. The first included stereotypes including drug users, homosexual men, and prostitutes. The second being the general perception that everyone is at risk.

Stereotypical perceptions

Given that young adults are noted for not being able to identify their own risk for HIV and STDs, participants were asked to describe who they considered being the most likely to contract HIV. While a number of types of people were mentioned, strikingly most perceptions focused on popular stereotypes. As Conrad identified, "I think it is just because that is how it has been portrayed in the media. Early on it was always seen with homosexuals. I think it's not so much the case for younger generations but more so the older ones." Ashley also commented on how some groups, such as homosexuals, and others were at an increased risk,

"I feel like gay people are the most at risk. I mean thinking about the epidemic it has greatly affected them. Therefore, that is one community that has really been affected. The other being Africa. So yeah those two groups need to worry." When Kayla was asked who was at risk for HIV she remarked, "Any homosexual dude, and pretty much all African Americans in general."

Finally, while Sophie did draw attention to another common group, drug users, she was the first and only participant to identify social economic status and education as determinants,

> I guess that is a tough one. I do not want to say drug users. I guess anyone who has multiple partners. But like a group specific I would say low-income areas. Going back to the fact that maybe they do not have the money to buy new drug equipment. Or have the education, or the money, or funding to get birth control or condoms and stuff like that. They would be the most at risk.

Statements such as these draw clear attention to the fact that HIV is not discussed in a manner that teaches viewers the facts about HIV. It may be understood that HIV does not pick and choose who it infects, but for some of the participants the impression remains that only some groups are at risk.

Everyone, but Me

The second population participants identified remained far broader; this being anyone, as well as anyone who has unprotected sex. While only mentioned by two participants, the idea that "everyone" is at risk was presented. Far more common, however, was the notion that anyone having unsafe sex would be at risk. Holly noted, "Risk is anything unprotected. So if you have unsafe sex you are at risk. It's pretty simple." Specifically taking note of what unsafe sex meant, Kathryn stated, "Anyone who doesn't use condoms is having unsafe sex." Yet while many participants agreed that everyone engaging in unprotected sex could be at risk, the fact remained that many were unable, or unwilling, to see themselves as someone at risk.

When asked if they felt they were at risk only three felt they "might be." The remainder finding comfort in either being married, no longer having sex, or as Anna identified have a partner they "know and can trust." Feeling that they "know" their partners decreases the need to discuss topics such as STDs and HIV.

College Students' Risk for HIV

Shifting the conversation to the exploration of peers' risk for HIV participants shared a strikingly different perception. Resoundingly, all of the participants felt their peers were at risk. One example found was Mark. When asked if he was at risk he replied, "Me, no. I am always safe." When asked about his peers he commented, "YES (college students are at risk), I feel college students are usually the dumb people who drink, party, and have sex, and forget the most important thing, using protection. Many times even though we are college students, we act before we think." Mark was not alone in the perception that college students were at risk due to a lack of thinking. Kristina argues that one's risk for HIV is far simpler: "If you are just not thinking about what you are doing, that puts you at risk." With this in mind Kristina was asked if she thought there were any groups of people she felt were at an increased risk because of this "lack of thinking"; to this she replied, "Ha, like college students." Kristina continued pointing out that overall college students were at risk for HIV because of the fact they are "Well they are lazy, alcoholics, and not thinking about what they are doing and their actions. They just don't think about the repercussions or diseases and stuff." Yet, Kristina was not alone; many of the participants indicated that college students in general seem to share a lack of awareness or concern for HIV or any disease.

Building onto the perception that college students do not think about their actions, Anna notes, "(College students) don't think they need to use protection. They think, 'Oh I know this person.'" Anna further explains, that college students feel that they only sleep with people they "know and can trust." Susan also shared "I know my partners and I don't pick up strange guys. These are people I know from school. So I know I will be fine." Disagreeing with the point that college students "know their partners" Ben described his experience attending college parties, "I have been to a few house parties and had to leave. People were having girls sleeping with everyone and they were all drunk and not thinking." Although Ben was the only one to comment on the casual sex that has occurred at parties a number of participants drew attention to the problem of drinking and making sound decisions.

Numerous students mentioned that drinking can impinge on a student's ability to think about preventive methods thus supporting a wealth of scholarship on the issue (e.g., Boone & Lefkowitz, 2004). Supporting this research Heather mentions that "at this time in our lives" college students are not thinking about HIV. She articulated,

> Unfortunately, at this time in our lives, probably the furthest thing from our minds is HIV. It is probably for the typical college student drinking Thursday, Friday, and Saturday Night. Finding this party and someone to hook up with,

> finals as they are quickly approaching, for the studious ones it's focusing on grades and occasional having fun and letting off steam.

Although much of their risky behavior is attributed to drinking, Audrey felt that the amount college students drank does not totally explain their behavior. Instead, she notes that, more often than not, two of the barriers to healthy behaviors come into play,

> I do not think they (college students) have any kind of forethought. I think that even when they are not drinking. I think they are aware but they still put themselves at risk. . . . The message is out there it is just making the connection for yourself. There seems to be a disconnect.

This notion that college lacked "any kind of forethought" also connects to the lack of thinking noted by other participants but her comment also identifies the disconnect college students feel in terms of their risk. In a similar manner, Ginger made note of the fact that besides drinking and the use of other drugs a major reason college students use protection was due to a lack of awareness. Related when asked directly if she felt college students would be at risk, Kayla replied, "No. Not really." Later on in the interview Kayla argued that for college students HIV is "just so far off" and not something she or her friends feel they need to worry about. Additionally, she noted, "We never talk about it. In addition, even like STDs are way more common and that is something to worry about. But none of us worry about HIV." Others also echoed the notion that STDs were a concern, but not HIV. Susan said, "Well maybe we are not at risk for HIV but definitely for STDS." As a result it appears two different disconnects seem to be occurring. The first of which is the identification of HIV as an STD and the second being the ability to see themselves as a population at risk.

HIV Is Too Taboo

Speaking to why HIV is not shown as a problem in the United States, Audrey identified major differences between the United States and her home country of Brazil. She explained that in her country sex messages are "everywhere "and talking about sex was always a natural thing, "Like we talk about safe sex like people talk here about getting a flu shot." Yet nearly all the other participants specifically noted that in the United States talking about safe sex has always been a "taboo" topic. Before HIV, and topics surrounding the idea of safe sex, can be health topics young people can actively think about, the frame surrounding them must be challenged.

Participants felt that, in general, talking about HIV or STDs, "makes people uncomfortable." Nearly all participants explained that the reason people and the media do not talk about HIV is because it's a taboo topic. Dorothy explained, "It's one of those taboo things." Similarly Sophie mentioned, "It's too taboo and will make people feel uncomfortable." Kristina added, "It's difficult. It is just not something you want to talk about. You do not want to talk about death or body issues. Dying. That is a taboo topic and HIV causes death." Sex has always been a topic that parents, teachers, and pastors alike have feared talking about. As a result this fear may be passed on to their children, who are not engaging in the behaviors that shall not be discussed.

Yet while many find that HIV is a taboo topic, many commented that other sexual topics are covered at great length. Ali explains, "I think people are drawn more to the teen pregnancy topics. So HIV just gets pushed to the wayside." Furthering this idea Austin notes, "I think it is just becoming a common thing," indicating that maybe HIV does not need to be discussed given that "everyone knows about it, so why focus on it?" Although teen pregnancy is the result of unprotected sex, the "sexiness" of it has allowed for multiple shows and movies to attract a great deal of attention. However, this has never been the case for HIV or STDs.

TRANSPORTATION INTO TELEVISION NARRATIVES

Transportation theory describes the process of how audiences are emotionally and psychologically transported into a media persona's world (Brown 2011). Therefore, if transportation into an HIV narrative is to be achieved, shows must be found to present the topic in a probable manner. Additionally, it is argued that the deeper a viewer transports into a show the more they will recall, given the level of involvement one shares with the characters (Brown, Childers, & Waszak 1990; Newcomer 2014; Rubin et al. 1985). To get at this the researcher evaluated the level of recall the participant had as well as their comments regarding how realistic they felt shows that talked about HIV are.

Level of Recall

While all the participants were selected because they reported being able to recall a show that discussed the issue of HIV, many could not provide details about what they saw. Many discussed medical situations where a character had gone to the hospital for a "mysterious" illness, or was sick and dying. However, they were not able to recall how the patient contracted HIV. When the participants recalled seeing a show the researcher had analyzed, additional questions were asked targeted at details as a means of assisting the recall process. For example, as while Sophie could recall that the girls in the show *Sex and the City* discussed testing, all that was noted was that during the conversations each of the friends stated they had been tested. To this the researcher asked who the character was that brought the topic into conversation. Initially identifying the wrong character Sophie asked the researcher about the hair color of the one she named and quickly corrected her choice. Additionally, she was asked what she could remember of the test. Unfortunately, while the show did offer a complete testing experience, Sophie was only able to recall that the character tested negative. Only a few of the participants could recall episodes where characters talked openly about testing for HIV. Yet as with Sophie the other participants were only able to recall that the characters tested negative.

Interestingly, while many of the participants were unable to provide details of the shows that discussed the issue of HIV, many could not provide details about movies that had shared this theme. Regardless of how long ago they had seen it more details were offered of who the characters were, how they contracted HIV, as well as how this impacted their lives. One example of this was Ben who recalled, "Well the one that always comes to mind is Tom Hanks from *Philadelphia*. I remember that movie and that he played a character that had HIV and the legal battle, the way they treated him, the way it destroyed his life." Along with *Philadelphia* other popular movies mentioned and discussed included *Rent*, *MILK*, *Gia*, as well as mentions of various Lifetime movies and documentaries. The ability for participants to transport into these movies may be occurring in part because movies are longer and would be all-encompassing. However, another consideration is the ability for viewers to see HIV being shown in a real way.

The Reality of HIV

In addition to being asked what they could recall, participants were also asked if they felt that these shows were realistic. In many cases the answer varied from "absolutely not" to as Audrey states, "it's somewhat realistic . . . but not really." When asked what she meant by this Audrey explained, "There is no sense of urgency. It has a sense of distancing. It's like, 'Oh look this person needs to get tested.' As if we don't all have to. So in many ways it tokenizes it." Later, the interview returned to the issue of television shows "tokenizing" the issue of HIV and explained that by doing so the media "misses the chance they have to teach. They have your attention but they don't talk enough."

Beth also commented on the fact that shows seem to be missing opportunities to educate viewers, "Shows seem to be just reinforcing people's fears and they do not take the time to look up the facts. They just watch these shows and think that is who and what it is. . . . Shows just dramatize the whole situation and that is what people believe." Additionally, Beth pointed out, "Shows like *Dateline* go a good job. But other shows I do not think so. I think it is used for a dramatic effect and it does not help. It just adds to the stigma of the whole thing." By adding to this stigma surrounding HIV, viewers may learn that only some groups are at risk for HIV, which could explain why so many stereotypical groups were mentioned by participants when asked who was at risk.

In a similar vein, Mark also took note of the way television media seems to miss the opportunity to connect with audiences, "I feel like shows should use real people that have the disease. I feel like this is a strong way to connect with any audience. Also the show would need to be able to show all the negative sides to HIV such as what it does to your body and the possible end results. I just do not think people see the scary side anymore. It is just not a big deal." Other participants also commented that through the use of reality shows viewers would not be more likely to watch the show, but given the "realness" of the characters they may be more likely to feel a sense of connection.

VIEWER IDENTIFICATION WITH CHARACTERS

Once an individual perceives similarities with HIV-positive individuals, he or she is increasingly more likely to personalize their own risk of HIV (Crowell & Emmers-Sommer, 2000). Therefore, in order for viewers to learn from television narratives they must be able to connect with characters and see themselves within the shows. Unfortunately, for many of the participants the portrayal of HIV was either found to be unrealistic or appeared to only focus on stereotypical groups.

An Unrealistic Portrayal of HIV

As postulated by Cohen (2001), a viewer's identification to a character relies on both emotional and cognitive processes to which the viewer forgets about his or her own reality. However, one problem noted by participants was that in general fictional shows are seen as over-dramatizations and therefore regardless of the topic may be perceived as being less realistic.

Ben states,

> No (they are not realistic), TV never shows the consequences. They make light of it or use it to get your attention and then move on. You know, they show someone getting pregnant or contract something and it's a joke. They never tell the story of the person who didn't have safe sex and got something. It's always a joke or everything ends up working out. But that is not reality. So no, they do not express, portray or show consequences in a realistic way.

Commenting on the impact real characters could have, Mark said, "I feel a show should use real people who have the disease. I feel it will be a strong way to connect to the audience. Also the show would need to show all the negative sides to HIV such as what it can do to your body." Another issue participants mentioned was the proliferation for sex to be used to sell, and that focusing on consequences would not be perceived as sexy enough to retain viewers. Ginger also addressed the concern that shows she has seen have neglected to show how HIV could actually impact one's life or who was at risk for HIV:

> I think they need to cut out the fluff. Like really show you how terrible life can get or how it affects your life. Also show that it was possible for anybody to get it if you're not having safe sex or using condoms or doing what you are supposed to be doing to prevent it. I feel like they just make it seem like only some people can get it. And it was a lot more like I feel I was more aware of it when it seemed like anyone could get it and not just these people. And I guess that it seems like it is only some people get it which I do not know.

By showing young heterosexual adults engaged in risky behavior without consequences of STDs or HIV also perpetuates normative behavior. Young adults are often found to feel that they are not at risk for anything and if shows are going to offer the social model of the consequence of unsafe sexual behavior then greater attention will need to be paid to who is shown being subject to the consequence.

With this in mind, it should be noted that television has long been criticized for portraying unrealistic depictions of health-risk behaviors (Ward & Friedman 2006). As a result, there is the potential for these depictions to be accepted as the norm, thus influencing viewers' perceptions and behaviors. Within the current study the majority of participants were only able to recall HIV-positive characters who were drug users, homosexuals, or dying. Scott comments, "I feel like they need to do a better job of not just portraying some demographics. Not only showing gays but also straight people."

Perpetuation of Stereotypes

When looking at who college students recall seeing in the television narratives only one noted seeing a character that could possibly offer some point of similarity, however, this character was a high school teen. Anna states, "I have seen a wide range. Especially on Lifetime. They try to show more "normal" people. I saw, the one I just mentioned was a teenager and it was her first time having sex and she got it. Otherwise I have seen everyone, homosexuals, promiscuous, and prostitutes." Similar to other participants she also commented on the overly dramatic and less realistic ways HIV has been portrayed. Anna noted, "I think (shows on television) are getting there. But they still seem like they are not giving the information. They still lead people to believe it is only homosexuals and prostitutes. It's very few shows where you can see the "average" person getting it.

Yet when asked if she could think of any examples where the "average" person was shown with HIV she stated, "No. That is a problem. Maybe in a documentary but nothing in the mainstream."

During Kristina's interview, she highlighted the potential problem with focusing on these types of characters stating,

> I mean I guess I do kind of think about it (her risk for HIV) and I am like well yeah I guess I should be more careful and stuff. But like since they do show it more with gay males then I do not think about it as much for myself. You know like I am not gay. But I like people, so maybe I could have been with a person who liked other people. I guess they could have been gay and not told me.

Both Kristina and Anna address the feeling that the way HIV has been represented on television is not done so in a way that they feel a connection to.

Due to the ongoing stigma surrounding HIV it seems logical that young adults, or anyone for that matter, would not want to self-identify as being at risk for HIV. Ryan points out that, in shows such as *CSI: NY*, "HIV is shown being transmitted through needles and stuff like that. Or else it is like this taboo type of thing. They do not really refer to it. It is kind of this tainted kind of image. But they never really talk about what happened or things like that. But I think shows like CSI could talk more about how people got it." When asked what he meant by HIV being a "tainted" topic he replied, "You're dirty if you have it. And normally people get it some way you wouldn't want people to know about." It is this kind of mind frame that leads to the perpetuation of stigma and ignorance. While HIV is preventable if proper action is taken, there are also the cases where partners and spouses may have contracted the virus prior to the relationship and simply didn't know.

Ben also took time to discuss how many of today's shows neglect to teach viewers about HIV. Fervently he argued, "People don't like consequences. So why would they watch a show that would include them? TV producers know that." However, as found within the current interviews, viewers seem to have learned that because there are no consequences for the "everyday normal person" and only consequences for the "dirty" and "tainted" people, people they would not associate with, they would not be at risk and therefore have learned that they do not need to identify themselves as being at risk for HIV.

WHAT THE VIEWER'S PERCEPTIONS TEACH US

The aim of this chapter was to supplement the current knowledge and understanding of how television narratives about HIV impede the ability for college students to accurately perceive their risk. In doing so, I extend the conversation of media effects by illuminating ways in which observational learning may be dependent upon a viewer's' identification with the show's characters. Relying upon rhetorical analysis, the earlier chapters not only identified how HIV was presented, but also dissected the content, characters, and situations used to frame the topic of HIV. As a result, valuable dichotomies in which this illness is socially constructed were revealed.

Overall what the interviews teach us is that although the rhetorical analysis indicated two primary didactic narratives, normal and stigmatized, only the stigmatized narratives are reflected in the perceptions of these college students. Results therefore indicate that identification and transportation with mediated HIV narratives do impact viewers' perceptions of risk and behavior. Unfortunately, for college students the lesson learned from these narratives is that only certain groups are affected by HIV, and they are not one of those groups. Ultimately, while it is clear entertainment-education can be an effective tool for educating viewers about health topics, a number of challenges for using television as a tool for modifying the perceptions of risk for HIV remain.

Identification with the Narratives

A viewer's ability to connect with the characters of a show, referred to as identification, has been found to play a vital role in developing perceptions surrounding an issue. It is also argued that a common barrier to a behavioral change is the lack of identification between the health issue and the individual (Moyer-Gusé 2008). If a viewer is able to make a connection with the characters of a show, or obtain perceived similarity, they will also increase their perception of vulnerability.

For the participants of the current chapter identification did not happen. Various types of characters were found to be present in television narratives including people with a variety of sexual orientations and racial backgrounds, however, little variation of age could be seen or recalled by participants. As a result, participants reported a feeling of disconnection between themselves and HIV, given that they were unable to see how characters were like them. The characters they could recall were mainly from stereotypical populations. As a consequence, participants did not gain a sense of perceived similarity with the characters and therefore missed the potential identification with a character, increasing their perceived invulnerability to contracting HIV.

Perceived similarity and identification with a character is thought to enhance the persuasive effects of entertainment-education content by increasing a viewer's perceived vulnerability (Moyer-Gusé 2008). This tendency is sometimes labeled as an "optimism bias"—the belief that one is unique, invulnerable, and that negative consequences of risky behavior will not affect him or her (Goossens, Beyers, Emmen, & Van Aken 2002; Moyer-Gusé & Nabi 2011). For the college students, the mentality of "it can't happen to me" was dominant. As a few of the participants noted, many of their peers share this perception given that they never personally see people like them having HIV.

Beyond feeling invulnerable to HIV, for nearly all the participants identification with HIV was impossible given their perceptions were that only "social deviants" are used to address the topic. Specifically, participants identified people living with HIV as being sick, dying, homosexual, highly promiscuous, dirty, or drug users. As a result, it is of no surprise that with most of the participants focusing their perceptions on general stereotypes, they would not be able to see themselves being at risk. This focus on stereotypes and "social deviants" also explains why throughout the interviews, many of the participants remarked feeling disconnected from characters on television. Generally speaking, viewers rarely will want to identify with the villain of a story or the social outcast. Yet in many of the shows HIV is not only referred to as "a punishment for past mistakes" but it is only shown impacting characters whose behaviors are often looked down upon. As a result, viewers will seek to identify the ways in which they are different from the characters. Therefore, the opportunity for gaining a sense of personal identification is lost.

Mediated narratives could allow for this connection to be made, however, the characters and situations used within current episodes fail to make a connection between college students and HIV. For example, participants commonly recounted the characters shown living with HIV (including doctors, lawyers, or mothers) coming to the hospital because they are sick and dying. In these situations, both the characters as well as the situation misses the opportunity to connect with young viewers. However, if episodes were able show HIV taking place in a college setting, or even including young adults in other settings, viewers may be able to see the similarities in the fact they do the same kinds of things. For instance, showing characters in college, talking with friends before a party or in the union about the weekend before. As a result, the opinion that "this doesn't happen to people like me" is challenged because there is the opportunity to finally see that character being similar to themselves.

Without a sense of personal identification and similarity viewers will not be able to increase their level of vulnerability. While many participants stated that anyone who has unprotected sex is at risk, something researchers have found college students frequently do (Baldwin & Baldwin, 2000), they could not personally identify as being a person at risk. As such it becomes clear that little to no level of vulnerability is maintained by young adults. Comments such as "HIV doesn't happen to us" and it's "not something we think about" not only highlight the lack for personal invulnerability, but it also offers an explanation for the lack of correspondence between an individual's knowledge of potential negative consequences of a behavior, such as having unprotected sex, and actually engaging in that behavior.

Transportation into Narratives

Transportation is concerned with the immersion of individuals within narrative content. The result of such transportation is that the viewer will connect with the narrative to the extent that it might change their beliefs, attitudes, and behaviors. As Moyer-Gusé (2008) points out, transportation should reduce a viewer's desire to argue with the messages presented. This is due to the viewer being swept up in the narrative and thus not motivated to argue story points (Fransen, Smit, & Verlegh 2015; Green & Brock 2000; Knowles & Linn, 2004; Slater & Rouner 2002). One barrier to achieving transportation lies in the reliance for viewers to identify with characters. It is argued that for learning through television narratives to occur viewers need to share a connection with the characters of a show, or gain perceived similarity. This increased engagement will then stimulate the ability to be transported into the show.

Based on the characters and situations used to discuss HIV in mediated narratives college students have remained unconnected with characters and have only gained support for their previously held perceptions. Research has maintained that people are more motivated to voluntarily expose themselves to programs and messages that support their current views (Tsfati & Cappella 2003). As a result, when a message supports preexisting perceptions of an issue it would be easier for participants to recall the message presented within an episode. This suggests that previously held beliefs of the audience have a significant impact on the level of trust they will have in the messages that are presented. For many of the participants in this study, regardless of the show, characters, or themes presented, only aspects of the show that supported previously held beliefs were recalled. Such beliefs included who would get HIV as well as the modes of contraction.

To this point Moyer-Gusé (2008) identifies that parasocial interaction with a character displaying counternormative behavior would enhance the persuasive effects of entertainment-education content by changing viewers' perceived norms. Moyer-Gusé (2008) states, "an individual's perception of norms surrounding a given behavior can also lead to resistance of a persuasive message" (419). Therefore, if a risky behavior, such as casual unprotected sex, is perceived as normative, information about the potential negative consequences of such behavior can be discounted through the use of strategic E-E programming. To this Gerrard, Gibbons, Benthin, Hessling, (1996) argue that individuals may engage in "false consensus"—normalizing one's risky behavior by claiming that "everyone" does it. For college students this occurs through not only watching peers within the college setting but also the numerous characters on television engaging in risky behavior without facing any consequences. As a result, entertainment-education programing will need to more accurately portray consequences for various ages and backgrounds. Doing so would not only increase the likelihood for a viewer to identify personal vulnerability, but the inclusion of consequences may also improve outcome expectancies

In one particular case, previously held perceptions appeared to color the participant's recollection of what happened within a narrative. Ashley spoke about the episode of *Nip/Tuck* where Christian has to be tested for HIV. In the episode he does test for HIV, however, in the end the redemption narrative comes to fruition and he finds out that he is not HIV positive. However, as Ashley recalls, "He finally gets what he deserves when he finds out he does have it." Not only does her comment imply HIV is a punishment for behaviors, a common thread in the shows, but she missed the ending where he does not receive a positive test.

Ashley's example draws attention to an important implication when examining television media effects on viewers' perception, this being the idea of inertia. Defined by Knowles and Linn (2004), inertia is the notion that individuals prefer not to change their attitudes, behaviors, and beliefs, and individuals will strive to maintain their previously held attitude systems. This results in selective avoidance of arguments that contradict one's existing beliefs and attitudes. For Ashely, risk for HIV is defined as "having multiple sexual partners and not really using protection." As a result, while she may have viewed the ending of the show where Christian finds out he is HIV negative, because of his sexual history on the show, she modified the ending to meet her previous impressions. Accordingly, while healthy conversations about HIV do occur every once in a while, until the normalization of talking about HIV, STDs, condoms, and safe sex practices is common practice, selective avoidance will remain a dominant practice. Overall, if Ashley had been able to identify with Christian in a more personal manner, research argues she would have been able to overcome inertia, and therefore enhancing her ability to transport into a show.

SUMMARY

Overall participants in the study subsequent to the HIV on Television analysis exhibited a disconnection in terms of their perception of their personal risk for HIV. Participants equally noted the media's lack of attention to HIV as a domestic issue. Beyond the lack of discussion surrounding the prevalence of HIV in the United States, participants also identified the inability for people to talk about sexually related topics. Additionally, these results provide a view, while limited, into the ways participants have been transported into the shows and movies they have seen. Finally, and of greatest concern, participants generally felt a lack of connection with people who are living with HIV. Partly this could be due to the lack of involvement or identification with the characters. However, it could also be explained by the larger lessons mediated narratives have taught.

NOTE

1. Pseudonyms are used for all interviewees in order to maintain their anonymity.

4

Stay Tuned for Clips of Next Season

Chapter Ten

Overcoming the Barriers and Moving Forward

Since the first report of the mysterious illness a great deal of knowledge about HIV and AIDS has been gained. Yet, regardless of advancements in knowledge, medical treatments, and government programs over 40,000 new infections are seen each year. People know facts and can recite the risks, yet intervention is still needed. The type of education required is not fact or risk driven, but on perception and stigma. For the 35 years fear of the punishment of HIV has continued to haunt characters, and the only real evolution was the slow return back to only talking about HIV in the gay populations.

Through this book a mediated history of HIV has been presented. Speaking out from the screen these narratives have potentially provided the only HIV education for two generations of viewers. However, the lessons taught have not remained consistent. The first generation learned to first fear HIV and anyone who might have it. This generation also received a mixed message in terms of whether or not this illness was a punishment. Countless shows fought against this perspective; however, when you look closely at who receives a positive test, and the bodies used to bring the storyline into play, it is easy to see a common theme. Those that look different from most viewers and are engaging in behaviors considered less than socially acceptable are the ones being punished. Early narratives presented HIV in strategic manners: embedding facts, models for peer conversations, and dispelling common misperceptions. Today's generation of viewers learns HIV is no big deal. In fact, HIV is so common that it can even be considered great material for a joke. In the past five years when a show included the topic of HIV, seven of every ten mentions used HIV as some form of punchline. This is not to say that jokes about HIV were completely absent from the mouths of previous characters, but today's joke seems to have much sharper teeth.

Modern narratives are no longer created in partnership with outside organizations, and truth be told facts are not what is needed today. Today viewers need to see themselves at risk. They need to see that everyone is at risk. HIV has never discriminated who it affected, yet according to television only some groups need to be concerned. While it is true some populations do see larger percentages of infection, and some behaviors do place people at higher risk, the fact of the matter is anyone can become infected. Until all walks of life are able to identify personal risk, the epidemic will continue.

This book's title presents HIV as popular culture's epidemic because it is my opinion that it is because of the way HIV has been framed and discussed in the media that has largely impacted perceptions. Unless a viewer is mid-twenties, white, and straight it is possible they will never see a person living with HIV who looks like them; which will almost certainly not occur on television. Therefore, on an individual level, viewers will be hit or miss in seeing a character they can identify with, and observe. If and when a character is identified, given the common theme of redemption the audience's primary lesson will be "see, everything turned out OK." Thus, no need to be tested, even though the show said they should. The lessons of HIV in mediated narratives have not only failed to provide consistent characters to appeal to a wide demographic, but more so by employing the comic and redemption frames HIV has been portrayed in such a way that justifies a lack of personal risk perception. To make matters worse, most of the narratives have encouraged if not perpetuated the stigma so many fought to break down in the 80s.

The early messages taught viewers that AIDS was not a punishment, it didn't only affect gay populations, and that everyone (even kids) were at risk. Today, HIV is a joke. A quick line or character tossed in to provide added drama. Today, given the cancelation of HBO's *Looking*, only one HIV-positive character is currently shown in a primetime show. And with nearly 10 other central characters in *How to Get Away with Murder* the HIV storyline will be given one, maybe two, mentions a season. According to America's television screens HIV is either a thing of the past, or an issue for other countries. That is until it's World AIDS Day, or when a popular celebrity comes out as living with the virus. Even then, depending on the celebrity, it might not even be "that surprising."

Given Charlie Sheen's wild past involving drugs and women the general public was less shocked by the news, and more concerned about how many people he would have given it to. In a 2015 interview with *Good Morning America*, Sheen explains that, thanks to the medications, he is feeling great and is "better than others. But, but most days are pretty frickin' cool." Sheen also states that he feels he is now "carrying the torch, for a lot of folks out there that are suffering from the same thing." Regardless of whether HIV-positive folk want Sheen as their torchbearer, the fact is his name remains well known. Audiences are now yet again shown that certain behaviors including drugs, sex with multiple women (and possibly some men), prostitution may result in HIV contraction. Thus, Sheen can be put up as the scapegoat and order can be maintained by pointing to him as the reminder for what not to do. In order to see less Charlie Sheens and less HIV as a whole, the perceptions that HIV and talking about sex in general are taboo need to be ruptured.

Regardless of how realistic a show is, or how similar a viewer is to the character one fact remains, talking about the prevention of HIV and STDs is perceived as a taboo topic. Seen as personal matter, talking about sex is a socially sensitive topic often only deemed appropriate to discuss when referring to creating a child. Society as a whole has established norms, commonly religiously based, about what is appropriate and moral regarding sex. Sex inside marriage, great. Sex for pleasure, sin. Sex to sell a pair of jeans, brilliant. Sex between two characters in a show with a condom, shameful and cannot be shown on television. These hypocrisies in how sex is discussed therefore lead to a country full of confused, uneducated, and unprepared audience members.

To be fair, television narratives have come a long way in terms of talking about sex, shifting from showing married couples sleeping in separate beds, to near strangers or coworkers finding the nearest coat room for a "quickie." Yet, many of the participants in chapter nine spoke directly about how afeard and taboo they felt portrayals of HIV, and condoms, on television remain to be. As a result, it is clear that simply showing people talking about HIV, in attempts to normalize the topic, doesn't work. Thus, until HIV, and other sexually related topics, are not seen as taboo and difficult topics to talk about with peers, partners, as well as doctors, then it seems unlikely that any amount of HIV narratives within television will ever overcome the perception that sex is not something one discusses.

Realistically, the best means of breaking down the taboo of talking about sex from a health perspective is the conversation with a medical provider. Conversations with medical providers are found to provide vital opportunities to offer STI and HIV counseling and testing for overall improved sexual health (Lanier, Castellanos, Barrow, Jordan, Caine, & Sutton 2014). Regardless of reason for the medical visit, discussions between patients and providers are a proactive strategy for increasing routine STI and HIV testing. When comprehensive sexual histories are obtained, providers are able to assess patients' behavioral risks, offer STI and/or HIV testing, and provide effective risk-reduction counseling (Nusbaum, & Hamilton 2002; Wimberly, Hogben, Moore-Ruffin, Moore, & Fry-Johnson 2006).

Unfortunately, routine sexual history taking is not a common practice among health care providers (Nusbaum, & Hamilton 2002; Wimberly, Hogben, Moore-Ruffin, Moore, & Fry-Johnson 2006). Despite the 2006 CDC recommendations, providers in healthcare settings are to perform routine

HIV testing for patients aged 13–64 years; research has found that less than 40 percent of medical providers are following the guidelines (Dorell, Sutton, Oster, et al. 2011; Wong, Jordan, Malebranche, DeLaitsch, Abravanel, Bermudez, Baugh 2013; Zheng, Yin, Suneja, Chou, & Arya 2014). Testing for HIV alone provides valuable prevention opportunities. Therefore, if a goal is to increase HIV and STI testing, showing characters in an episode engaged in a conversation where a medical provider speaks openly, frankly, and clearly about the test and risks of HIV, viewers may be less likely to avoid the topic the next time they themselves are in the doctor's office.

Starting with showing more medical providers on television engaged in open, non-judgment, discussions with patients about sexual health and prevention measures will not only help provide a script for the patient viewers, but also the providers themselves. Providers themselves are likely to feel uncomfortable broaching the topic for fear of accusing the patient of engaging in risky behaviors. Or they might share the feeling that only some populations need to be tested, and therefore why waste the resources. But with the estimation that only 50 percent of people living with HIV know their status, it is worth the test if it means diagnosis is found, and treatment can begin.

Beyond showing medical providers on television discussing sex, encouraging all patients to receive testing, the narrative structures themselves need updating. Messages are less likely challenged or resisted if the viewer is entertained. Yet that should be misconstrued as justification to make jokes about HIV. The fact is, *South Park* is wrong, we have not reached a time where HIV is funny. However, this is not to say that HIV narratives must only be dramatic. Comedy can be used as a conduit for the discussion, but HIV itself should not be the punchline. Many of the narratives have been criticized as being too close to an "after school special" and therefore easily dismissed. If anything, the long-standing understanding is that the less overtly persuasive a message is perceived to be, the more accepting receivers are to the influence (McGrane, Toth, & Allely 1990; Weinstein, Grubb, & Vautier 1986). With this in mind, HIV narratives need to be both informative and persuasive but the health message needs to be hidden under the guise of entertainment. HBO's *Looking* provided an important frame. Eddie was not defined by his HIV status; he simply was positive. When the situation deemed a discussion about testing, prevention, or disclosure it occurred organically.

The pace and realism of an HIV discussion is vital. The viewers interviewed in chapter nine felt that the only way to end the stigma related to HIV, as well as the perception that only certain groups are at risk for HIV, is for the discourse surrounding HIV and safe sex to become a normal part of society. These viewers noted that, often, the time they see HIV presented is in medical dramas, where the patient is sick and dying. Knowing that HIV is treatable and that the "visibly sick" stereotype is not the case for most of the people living with the virus today, many of the participants remarked that they wished television shows would do a better job of accurately depicting the everyday lives of someone living with HIV. In doing so, the viewers would learn not only that someone living with HIV is just like them, but also it would help break down the stigma that living with HIV means you are less than human.

One of the most interesting and consistent points drawn out by the viewers interviewed was that they nearly all agreed that one of the fastest ways to gain the attention of young adults is to include "real" people living with HIV into the shows they watched. Suggestions for characters on shows like *Keeping Up with the Kardashians* or *The Bachelor* to at the very least talk about testing for HIV or using condoms were specially noted. Participants argue that condoms would not have to be shown being used, but mentioned or shown on a table. By simply implying condoms would be used might help to increase the perception that this is a normal behavior. Additionally, the viewers felt that if more real people, especially young people, were shown living with HIV, then viewers would be better able to connect to the characters.

Bandura explains that "even people who are well informed on a health topic often err in their subjective appraisal of the extent to which they are putting themselves at risk" (3). As a result, unless viewers are able to see themselves at risk for HIV they are less likely to be motivated to alter their behaviors. Ultimately, popular culture's HIV only affects those needing to be punished. Therefore, a continued lack of personal connection to the characters in HIV narratives seems likely. Viewers will then remain unmotivated to seek testing or use protection. Why would they; they are not the one's at risk.

Until shows highlight the actual settings and characters that a wide variety of viewers, including young impressionable minds, can identify with, thus enhancing one's self-efficacy, the virus will continue to win. Pushing HIV back into the shadows, or continuing to exclusively show gay populations affected will only perpetuate stigma. Observations of realistic messages will prove incapable of affecting viewers' beliefs that they can and should regulate their own behavior.

When shows include health topics without strategically embedding accurate information, viewers may absorb inaccurate messages and lessons. As a result, shows incorporating health messages for the sake of drama risk unintentionally creating or reinforcing misperceptions, stereotypes, and stigma. At the same time when a message leaps of the screen and hits the viewer like an educational ruler across the hands the message will be dismissed. Both of these approaches mis-educate viewers about the consequences of risky behaviors and perpetuate stereotypes. Ultimately, over time more and more shows have missed the opportunity to illustrate HIV in a realistic and relatable manner. Those that do, are often cancelled, as was HBO's *Looking*.

Thus, yet another chance to break down the biggest barriers to HIV prevention, the ability to talk openly about sexual health, is taken away.

Although HIV is 100 percent preventable, until the narratives surrounding the virus evolve I fear the virus will remain. Knowledge, medications, and testing advancements are useless if people remain content in stages of pre-contemplation. Thinking to themselves, "I don't do that," "I'm not gay," "I've never done drugs," or "I would never share a needle," "My partner is clean." Convinced that only those that are deserving of punishment will contract the virus. As a result, if HIV is punishment, why would "I" want to be seen at a clinic? Why would a doctor mention testing to "me"? And finally, why should the government spend money to help "those" people?

From the beginning HIV has remained both directly and indirectly a political issue. Receiving countless reports giving warning of the epidemic, politicians held back on acknowledging AIDS, let alone directing money toward finding a cure. Possibly, the lack of response from the government was due to the behaviors themselves, or maybe it was because of populations HIV impacted. Either way the message early on implied that maybe HIV was killing off all the right people. Once public officials did start taking action all other aspects of the narrative were able to follow suit. Schools, though still limited by abstinence-only programs, began talking about HIV in health classes, and public health clinics nationwide were able to reach out and serve their communities. Additionally, global initiatives such as PEPFAR, George W. Bush's federal anti–HIV/AIDS foreign aid program began. Bush also established the Global AIDS Act of 2003. The Global AIDS Act becoming the single largest global health initiative targeting a single disease in history. Providing support for antiretroviral treatment for 7.7 million people, both directly and through technical support to partner countries.

Recognizing the importance of preventing HIV within the United States, President Obama took action quickly, signing the Ryan White Treatment Extension Act in October of 2009. This Act reauthorized the Ryan White HIV/AIDS Program; a program serving over 500,000, or approximately half, of all Americans living with HIV. A few months later the Obama administration took measures to help reduce HIV stigma and discrimination by lifting the entry ban for tourists and immigrants living with HIV. In July 2010, President Obama released the National HIV/AIDS Strategy detailing extensive backing for prevention programs, grants for further research, and support for those living with the virus. In July 2011, the National Institutes of Health (NIH) announced the preliminary results of the HIV Prevention Trial Network study 052, indicating that early initiation of antiretroviral treatment reduced the risk of transmitting HIV by 96 percent. Finally, in December 2011, President Obama declared that an AIDS-free generation was within reach.

That same year, then congressman Mike Pence began laying the groundwork for Indiana's own HIV outbreak, when the House passed his amendment to defund Planned Parenthood. A few years later in 2013, and now governor of Indiana, Scott County's one Planned Parenthood closed in the wake of public health spending cuts. Serving as the county's only HIV testing center, there was no longer a place for the county's 24,000 residents to get tested. A few years later Pence, who had been quoted as being morally opposed to needle exchanges, believing they promoted drug use, continued to actively work against HIV prevention by defunding needle exchange programs in the county. With nearly 20 percent of Scott County residents living below the poverty line, injection drugs remained a pubic health concern. Thus, it should be of no surprise that the county soon began seeing dangerous increases in new HIV infections.

Now serving as Vice President of the United States, Pence has reportedly taken a new stance on drug programs, however, he has remained steadfast on his opposition to the work of Planned Parenthood. Extending the views on HIV prevention the newest administration has already dismissed the members of a federal advisory council on HIV and AIDS. It is too soon to see what other HIV programs and initiatives will be hit, or killed, by this administration, but if history provides any indication, and the rise of infections seen in Indiana are any insight, it would appear the United States will not see an AIDS-free generation for decades to come.

Living in the United States today has convinced many that HIV is an issue of the 80s and in Africa. What was once a death sentence, is now nothing more than a chronic illness, "no big deal." Ultimately, the problem with these modes of thinking is not that people know less about HIV. Thanks to Google, the facts are searchable. The problem is, those that need to be searching have been convinced they don't need to. Those that need testing the most, are likely shamed into silence. After all, who would want to find out that they are in fact going to be punished for their actions?

Appendix A

SHOW LISTING

The following is a list of the shows analyzed for the book.

21 Jump Street
90210
A Different World
Always Sunny in Philadelphia
American Dad
Angels in America
Another World
Becker
The Best Years
Beverly Hills, 90210
Boston Legal
Brothers and Sisters
The Closer
Commander in Chief
CSI: NY
Dawson's Creek
Degrassi High
Designing Women
ER
Everwood
The Equalizer
Family Guy
General Hospital
Girlfriends

Go Toward the Light
Golden Girls
Grey's Anatomy
Half and Half
Hill Street Blues
Hollyoaks
Hotel
House, MD
How to Get Away with Murder
JAG
L.A. Law
Law and Order: SVU
The League
Life Goes On
Looking
Kids in the Hall
Melrose Place
Midnight Caller
Mr. Belvedere
Murder One
Neon Rider
Nip/Tuck
NYPD Blue
One on One
OZ
The Parkers
Picket Fences
Private Practice
Queer as Folk
Saturday Night Live
Scrubs
Seinfeld
Sex and the City
South Park
Star Trek: Enterprise
St. Elsewhere
Thirtysomething
Touched by an Angel
Without a Trace

Bibliography

21 Jump Street. "Cory and Dean Got Married." Episode number 21. Directed by Kim Manners. Written by Clifton Campbell. FOX (US), May 8, 1988.

Adefuye, Adedeji S., Titilayo C. Abiona, Joseph A. Balogun, and Mainza Lukobo-Durrell. "HIV sexual risk behaviors and perception of risk among college students: implications for planning interventions." *BMC public health* 9, no. 1 (2009): 281.

A Different World. "If I Should Die Before I Wake." Episode number 23. Directed by Debbie Allen.

Albarracín, Dolores, Penny S. McNatt, Wendy R. Williams, Tamara Hoxworth, Jonathan Zenilman, Ringo M. Ho, Fen Rhodes, C. Kevin Malotte, Gail A. Bolan, and Michael Iatesta. "Structure of outcome beliefs in condom use." *Health Psychology* 19, no. 5 (2000): 458.

Albert, Dustin, and Laurence Steinberg. "Judgment and decision making in adolescence." *Journal of Research on Adolescence* 21, no. 1 (2011): 211–224.

American Academy of Pediatrics. Sexuality, Contraception, and the Media: The Council on Communications and Media. *Pediatrics*, 126 (2010): 576–582. doi: 10.1542/peds.2010–1544

American College Health Association. American College Health Association National College Health Assessment Spring 2007 Reference Group Data Report. *Journal of American College Health, 561* (2007): 469–479.

American Dad!. "Max Jets." Episode number 11. Directed by Jennifer Graves. Written by Seth MacFarlane. TBS, February 10, 2013.

An Early Frost. Directed by John Erman. Universal City, CA: Universal Studios, 1985.

Asbeek Brusse, Elsbeth D., Marieke L. Fransen, and Edith G. Smit. "Educational storylines in entertainment television: audience reactions toward persuasive strategies in medical dramas." *Journal of Health Communication* 20, no. 4 (2015): 396–405. http://dx.doi.org/10.1080/10810730.2014.965365.

Ashenhurst, James R., Emily R. Wilhite, K. Paige Harden, and Kim Fromme. "Number of sexual partners and relationship status are associated with unprotected sex across emerging adulthood." *Archives of sexual behavior* 46, no. 2 (2017): 419–432.

Aubrey, Jennifer Stevens, Kristen Harrison, Leila Kramer, and Jennifer Yellin. "Variety versus timing: Gender differences in college students' sexual expectations as predicted by exposure to sexually oriented television." *Communication Research* 30, no. 4 (2003): 432–460.

Aubrey, Jennifer Stevens, Elizabeth Behm-Morawitz, and Kyungbo Kim. "Understanding the effects of MTV's 16 and pregnant on adolescent girls' beliefs, attitudes, and behavioral intentions toward teen pregnancy." *Journal of health communication* 19, no. 10 (2014): 1145–1160. http://dx.doi.org/10.1080/10810730.2013.872721.

Aubrey, Jennifer Stevens, and Siobhan E. Smith. "The impact of exposure to sexually oriented media on the endorsement of hookup culture: A panel study of first-year college students." *Mass Communication and Society* 19, no. 1 (2016): 74–101. http://dx.doi.org/10.1080/15205436.2015.1070875.

Bae, Hyuhn-Suhck. "Entertainment-education and recruitment of cornea donors: The role of emotion and issue involvement." *Journal of Health Communication* 13, no. 1 (2008): 20–36.

Baldwin, Janice I., and John D. Baldwin. "Heterosexual anal intercourse: an understudied, high-risk sexual behavior." *Archives of sexual behavior* 29, no. 4 (2000): 357–373.

Bandura, Albert. "Social foundations of thought and action." Englewood Cliffs, NJ (1986).

———. "Social cognitive theory of mass communication." *Media psychology* 3, no. 3 (2001): 265–299. http://dx.doi.org/10.1207/S1532785XMEP0303_03.

———. "Social cognitive theory for personal and social change by enabling media." *Entertainment-education and social change: History, research, and practice* (2004): 75–96.

Basen-Engquist, Karen. "Evaluation of a theory-based HIV prevention intervention for college students." *AIDS Education and Prevention* (1994).

Baxter, R., De Riemer, C., Landini, A., Leslie, L., & Singletary, M. (1985). "A content analysis of music videos." *Journal of Broadcasting & Electronic Media*, 29, 333–340.

Beck, Vicky, W. Pollard, and B. Greenberg. "Tune in for health: Working with television entertainment shows and partners to deliver health information for at-risk audiences." In *Presentation at the annual meeting of the American Public Health Association, Boston*. 2000.

Benoit, William L. "Beyond genre theory: The genesis of rhetorical action." *Communications Monographs* 67, no. 2 (2000): 178–192.

Besley, Tina. "Social education and mental hygiene: Foucault, disciplinary technologies and the moral constitution of youth." *Educational Philosophy and Theory* 34, no. 4 (2002): 419–433. doi:10.1111/j.1469–5812.2002.tb00517.x.

Biesecker, Barbara A. "Rethinking the Rhetorical Situation from within the Thematic of 'Différance.'" *Philosophy & rhetoric* (1989): 110–130.

Bleakley, Amy, Michael Hennessy, Martin Fishbein, and Amy Jordan. "How sources of sexual information relate to adolescents' beliefs about sex." *American Journal of Health Behavior* 33, no. 1 (2009): 37–48.

Boone, Tanya L., and Eva S. Lefkowitz. "Safer sex and the health belief model: Considering the contributions of peer norms and socialization factors." *Journal of Psychology & Human Sexuality* 16, no. 1 (2004): 51–68.

Boot, Inge, Jochen Peter, and Johanna MF van Oosten. "Impersonal sex orientation and multitasking influence the effect of sexual media content on involvement with a sexual character." *Media Psychology* 17, no. 1 (2014): 55–77. http://dx.doi.org/10.1080/15213269.2012.742358.

Borchers, Timothy. *Persuasion in the media age*. Waveland Press, 2012.

Brodie, Mollyann, Elizabeth Hamel, Lee Ann Brady, Jennifer Kates, and Drew E. Altman. "AIDS at 21: Media coverage of the HIV epidemic 1981–2002." *Columbia Journalism Review* 42, no. 6 (2004): A1.

Brothers & Sisters. "On the Road Again." Episode number 24. Directed by Ken Olin. Written by David Marshall Grant, Geoffrey Nauffts. ABC (US), May 16, 2010.

Brown, Jane D., Kim Walsh Childers, and Cynthia S. Waszak. "Television and adolescent sexuality." *Journal of Adolescent Health Care* 11, no. 1 (1990): 62–70.

Brown, Jane D., Kelly Ladin L'Engle, Carol J. Pardun, Guang Guo, Kristin Kenneavy, and Christine Jackson. "Sexy media matter: exposure to sexual content in music, movies, television, and magazines predicts black and white adolescents' sexual behavior." *Pediatrics* 117, no. 4 (2006): 1018–1027. doi: 10.1542/peds.2005–1406.

Brown, Jane D., Jeanne R. Steele, and Kim Walsh-Childers, eds. *Sexual teens, sexual media: Investigating media's influence on adolescent sexuality*. Routledge, 2001.

Brown, W. J. "Assessing processes of relational involvement with media personas: Transportation, parasocial interaction, identification and worship." In *National Communication Association conference, November*, pp. 15–19. 2011.

Brummett, Barry. "Burkean comedy and tragedy, illustrated in reactions to the arrest of John DeLorean." *Communication Studies* 35, no. 4 (1984): 217–227. http://dx.doi.org/10.1080/10510978409368191.

Buonanno, Milly. *The age of television: Experiences and theories*. Intellect Books, 2008.

Bui, Ngoc H. "Exploring similarity characteristics, identification, and parasocial interactions in choice of celebrities." Psychology of Popular Media Culture 6, no. 1 (2017): 21. http://dx.doi.org/10.1037/ppm0000082.

Burke, Kenneth. "The range of rhetoric." *A Rhetoric of Motives* (1950): 3–46.

Busselle, Rick W., and Bradley S. Greenberg. "The nature of television realism judgments: A reevaluation of their conceptualization and measurement." *Mass Communication & Society* 3, nos. 2–3 (2000): 249–268.

Cacioppo, John T., Wendi L. Gardner, and Gary G. Berntson. "The affect system has parallel and integrative processing components: Form follows function." *Journal of personality and Social Psychology* 76, no. 5 (1999): 839.

Collins, Rebecca L., Marc N. Elliott, Sandra H. Berry, David E. Kanouse, and Sarah B. Hunter. "Entertainment television as a healthy sex educator: The impact of condom-efficacy information in an episode of *Friends*." *Pediatrics* 112, no. 5 (2003): 1115–1121.

Carr, Jillian B., and Analisa Packham. "The Effects of State-Mandated Abstinence-Based Sex Education on Teen Health Outcomes." *Health Economics* (2016): 403–420. doi: 10.1002/hec.3315.

Caron, Sandra L., Clive M. Davis, William A. Halteman, and Maria Stickle. "Predictors of condom-related behaviors among first-year college students." *Journal of Sex Research* 30, no. 3 (1993): 252–259. http://dx.doi.org/10.1080/00224499309551709.

Centers for Disease Control and Prevention. "HIV in the United States: at a glance. 2013." *URL: http://www. cdc. gov/hiv/statistics/overview/ataglance. html [accessed 2016–0916] [WebCiteCache]* (2014).

Chandler, Daniel. "Children's Understanding of What is 'Real'on Television: a review of the literature." *Journal of Educational Media* 23, no. 1 (1997): 65–80.

Charmaz, Kathy. "Grounded Theory: objectivist and constructivist methods in Norman K. Denzin and Yvonne S. Lincoln (eds.) *Handbook of Qualitative Research*." United Kingdom: Sage Publications, 2000.

Civic, Diane. "College students' reasons for nonuse of condoms within dating relationships." *Journal of Sex & Marital Therapy* 26, no. 1 (2000): 95–105.

Commander in Chief. "First Scandal." Episode number 7. Directed by Daniel Attias. Written by Rod Lurie, Dee Johnson. ABC (US), November 8, 2005.

CSI: NY. "Heart of Glass." Episode number 16. Directed by David Jackson. Written by Bill Haynes, Pam Veasey. CBS, February 14, 2007.

Cohen, Jonathan. "Defining identification: A theoretical look at the identification of audiences with media characters." *Mass Communication & Society* 4, no. 3 (2001): 245–264. http://dx.doi.org/10.1207/S15327825MCS0403_01.

Collins, Rebecca L., Marc N. Elliott, Sandra H. Berry, David E. Kanouse, and Sarah B. Hunter. "Entertainment television as a healthy sex educator: The impact of condom-efficacy information in an episode of *Friends*." *Pediatrics* 112, no. 5 (2003): 1115–1121.

Clandinin, D. Jean, and F. Michael Connelly. "Narrative inquiry" (2000): 251–307.

Conrad, Peter, and Kristin K. Barker. "The social construction of illness key insights and policy implications." *Journal of health and social behavior* 51, no. 1 suppl (2010): S67–S79. doi: 10.1177/0022146510383495

Craig, David. "Calling Western Union: The cultural mission of television message movies." *Journal of Popular Film and Television* 42, no. 2 (2014): 60–70. http://dx.doi.org/10.1080/01956051.2013.805117.

Creswell, John W., and J. David Creswell. *Research design: Qualitative, quantitative, and mixed methods approaches*. Sage publications, 2017.

Crowell, Tara L., and Tara M. Emmers-Sommer. "Examining condom use self-efficacy and coping in sexual situations." *Communication Research Reports* 17, no. 2 (2000): 191–202.

d'Anjou, Leo. *Social movements and cultural change: the first abolition campaign revisited.* Transaction Publishers, 1996.

Davenport, L., LaRose, R. & Straubhaar, J. *Media Now - Understanding Media, Culture, and Technology* (6th ed.). Boston: Wadsworth, Cengage Learning, 2010.

Dawson's Creek. "Day Out of Days." Episode number 11. Directed by Robert Duncan McNeill. Written by Gina Fattore. The WB, January 15, 2003.

Degrassi High. "Bad Blood (1)." Episode number 1. Directed by Kit Hood. Written by Yan Moore. CBC (CA), September 3, 1990.

Degrassi High. "Bad Blood (2)." Episode number 2. Directed by Kit Hood. Written by Yan Moore. CBC (CA), September 3, 1990. Demmer, Craig, and Orazio Caroleo. "College students' perceptions of advances in HIV treatment and the need for safer sex practices." *Psychological Reports* 88, no. 2 (2001): 431–442.

Dilorio, Colleen, William N. Dudley, Johanna Soet, Joseph Watkins, and Edward Maibach. "A social cognitive-based model for condom use among college students." *Nursing research* 49, no. 4 (2000): 208–214.

Designing Women. "Killing All the Right People." Episode number 4. Directed by Harry Thomason. Written by Linda Bloodworth-Thomason. CBS, October 5, 1987.

Dorell, Christina G., Madeline Y. Sutton, Alexandra M. Oster, Felicia Hardnett, Peter E. Thomas, Zaneta J. Gaul, Leandro A. Mena, and James D. Heffelfinger. "Missed opportunities for HIV testing in health care settings among young African American men who have sex with men: implications for the HIV epidemic." *AIDS patient care and STDs* 25, no. 11 (2011): 657–664.

Dutta-Bergman, Mohan J. "Primary sources of health information: Comparisons in the domain of health attitudes, health cognitions, and health behaviors." *Health communication* 16, no. 3 (2004): 273–288. doi: 10.1207/s15327027hc1603_1.

Ellen, Jonathan M., Nancy Adler, Jill E. Gurvey, Susan G. Millstein, and Jeanne Tschann. "Adolescent condom use and perceptions of risk for sexually transmitted diseases: a prospective study." *Sexually transmitted diseases* 29, no. 12 (2002): 756–762. https://doi.org/10.1097/00007435–200212000–00004.

Everwood. "Just Like in the Movies." Episode number 9. Directed by Matt Shakman. Written by Rina Mimoun. The WB, November 17, 2003.

Everwood. "Controlling Interest." Episode number 12. Directed by Lev L. Spiro. Written by Michael Green. The WB, January 26, 2004.

Exner, Theresa M., David W. Seal, and Anke A. Ehrhardt. "A review of HIV interventions for at-risk women." *AIDS and Behavior* 1, no. 2 (1997): 93–124. doi:10.1023/B:AIBE.0000002972.61606.99.

Eyal, Keren. *The Role of Television Characters in Explaining Audience Sexuality.* Conference Papers—International Communication Association, 1. 2010.

Eyal, Keren, and Keli Finnerty. "The portrayal of sexual intercourse on television: How, who, and with what consequence?" *Mass Communication and Society* 12, no. 2 (2009): 143–169.

Eyal, Keren. "The effects of television drama shows on emerging adults' sexual attitudes and perceptions" (2000): 2414–2414.

Eyal, Tal, Nira Liberman, Yaacov Trope, and Eva Walther. "The pros and cons of temporally near and distant action." *Journal of personality and social psychology* 86, no. 6 (2004): 781.

Family Guy. "The Cleveland-Loretta Quagmire." Episode number 5. Directed by James Purdum. Written by Patrick Henry, Mike Henry (VI). FOX (US), June 12, 2005.

Farrar, Kirstie M. "Sexual intercourse on television: Do safe sex messages matter?" *Journal of Broadcasting & Electronic Media* 50, no. 4 (2006): 635–650. http://dx.doi.org/10.1207/s15506878jobem5004_4.

Freeman, Tierra M., Lynley H. Anderman, and Jane M. Jensen. "Sense of belonging in college freshmen at the classroom and campus levels." *The Journal of Experimental Education* 75, no. 3 (2007): 203–220. doi: 10.3200/JEXE.75.3.203–220.

Ferris, Amber L., Sandi W. Smith, Bradley S. Greenberg, and Stacy L. Smith. "The content of reality dating shows and viewer perceptions of dating." *Journal of Communication* 57, no. 3 (2007): 490–510.

Finnerty, Keli Lynn. *Risky sexual intercourse on entertainment television: Comparing audience responses to different types of negative consequence portrayals.* University of Arizona, 2007.

Fisher, Deborah A., Douglas L. Hill, Joel W. Grube, and Enid L. Gruber. "Sex on American television: An analysis across program genres and network types." *Journal of Broadcasting & Electronic Media* 48, no. 4 (2004): 529–553.

Fisher, Deborah A., Douglas L. Hill, Joel W. Grube, Melina M. Bersamin, Samantha Walker, and Enid L. Gruber. "Televised sexual content and parental mediation: Influences on adolescent sexuality." *Media Psychology* 12, no. 2 (2009): 121–147.

Fisher, Walter R. "Genre: Concepts and applications in rhetorical criticism." *Western Journal of Speech Communication* 44, no. 4 (1980): 288–299.

Flick, Uwe. Social representations in knowledge and language as approaches to a psychology of the social. In U. Flick (Ed.), *The psychology of the social.* Cambridge, England: Cambridge University Press, 1998.

Fontana, A., and J. H. Frey. "The Interview. From Structured Questions to Negotiated Text." *Handbook of Qualitative Research.* Norman K. Denzin and Yvonna S. Lincoln, eds. Thousand Oaks, CA: Sage Publications, 2000.

Foster, Diana Greene, Jenny A. Higgins, M. Antonia Biggs, Christy McCain, Sue Holtby, and Claire D. Brindis. "Willingness to have unprotected sex." *Journal of Sex Research* 49, no. 1 (2012): 61–68. doi: 10.1080/00224499.2011.572307.

Fransen, Marieke L., Edith G. Smit, and Peeter W. J. Verlegh. "Strategies and motives for resistance to persuasion: an integrative framework." *Frontiers in psychology* 6 (2015): 1201.

Galician, Mary-Lou. *Sex, love, and romance in the mass media: Analysis and criticism of unrealistic portrayals and their influence.* Routledge, 2004.

Gavin, Jeff. "Television teen drama and HIV/AIDS: The role of genre in audience understandings of safe sex." *Continuum: Journal of Media & Cultural Studies* 15, no. 1 (2001): 77–96. http://dx.doi.org/10.1080/713657765.

Gerrard, Meg, Frederick X. Gibbons, Alida C. Benthin, and Robert M. Hessling. "A longitudinal study of the reciprocal nature of risk behaviors and cognitions in adolescents: what you do shapes what you think, and vice versa." *Health Psychology* 15, no. 5 (1996): 344. http://dx.doi.org/10.1037/0278–6133.15.5.344.

Girlfriends. "Take This Poem and Call Me in the Morning." Episode number 12. Directed by Katy Garretson. Written by Lamont Ferrell, Norman Vance, Jr. UPN, January 6, 2003.

Girlfriends. "Howdy Partner." Episode number 13. Directed by Leslie Kolins-Small. Written by Tim Edwards. UPN, January 7, 2003.

Girlfriends. "Sex, Lies and Books." Episode number 16. Directed by Sheldon Epps. Written by Regina Y. Hicks. UPN, February 17, 2003.

Girlfriends. "The Pact." Episode number 19. Directed by Katy Garretson. Written by Michelle Marburger, Kevin Marburger, Michele Marburger. UPN, March 17, 2003.

Glik, Deborah, Emil Berkanovic, Kathleen Stone, Leticia Ibarra, Marcy Connell Jones, Bob Rosen, Myrl Schreibman, Lisa Gordon, Laura Minassian, and Darcy Richardes. "Health education goes Hollywood: Working with prime-time and daytime entertainment television for immunization promotion." *Journal of Health Communication* 3, no. 3 (1998): 263–282. http://dx.doi.org/10.1080/108107398127364.

The Golden Girls. "72 Hours." Episode number 19. Directed by Terry Hughes. Written by Richard Vaczy, Tracy Gamble. NBC, February 17, 1990.

Goffman, Erving. *Frame analysis: An essay on the organization of experience.* Harvard University Press, 1974.

———. *Stigma: Notes on the management of spoiled identity.* Simon and Schuster, 2009.

Goldman, Judith A., and Lisa L. Harlow. "Self-perception variables that mediate AIDS-preventive behavior in college students." *Health Psychology* 12, no. 6 (1993): 489.

Goossens, Luc, Wim Beyers, Mieke Emmen, and Marcel AG Van Aken. "The imaginary audience and personal fable: Factor analyses and concurrent validity of the 'new look' measures." *Journal of Research on Adolescence* 12, no. 2 (2002): 193–215. doi: 10.1111/1532–7795.00031.

Green, Melanie C., and Timothy C. Brock. "The role of transportation in the persuasiveness of public narratives." *Journal of personality and social psychology* 79, no. 5 (2000): 701.

Green, Melanie C., Timothy C. Brock, and Geoff F. Kaufman. "Understanding media enjoyment: The role of transportation into narrative worlds." *Communication Theory* 14, no. 4 (2004): 311–327. doi: 10.1111/j.1468–2885.2004.tb00317.x.

Greenberg, Bradley S., and Mark G. Woods. "The soaps: Their sex, gratifications, and outcomes." *Journal of Sex Research* 36, no. 3 (1999): 250–257. http://dx.doi.org/10.1080/00224499909551995.

Grey's Anatomy. "Piece of My Heart." Episode number 13. Directed by Mark Tinker. Written by Stacy McKee. ABC (US), May 1, 2008.

Grey's Anatomy. "The Time Warp." Episode number 15. Directed by Rob Corn. Written by Zoanne Clack. ABC (US), February 18, 2010.

Gunasekera, Hasantha, Simon Chapman, and Sharon Campbell. "Sex and drugs in popular movies: an analysis of the top 200 films." *Journal of the Royal Society of Medicine* 98, no. 10 (2005): 464–470.

Hart, Kylo-Patrick R. *The AIDS movie: Representing a pandemic in film and television.* Routledge, 2014.

Hauser, Philip M. "Movies, Delinquency and Crime." New York: Macmillan 320 (1933).

Hennessy, Michael, Amy Bleakley, Martin Fishbein, and Amy Jordan. "Validating an index of adolescent sexual behavior using psychosocial theory and social trait correlates." *AIDS and Behavior* 12, no. 2 (2008): 321–331. doi: doi:10.1007/s10461–007–9272–1.

"Health promotion by social cognitive means." *Health education & behavior* 31, no. 2 (2004): 143–164. https://doi.org/10.1177/1090198104263660.

Hether, Heather J., Grace C. Huang, Vicki Beck, Sheila T. Murphy, and Thomas W. Valente. "Entertainment-education in a media-saturated environment: Examining the impact of single and multiple exposures to breast cancer storylines on two popular medical dramas." *Journal of health communication* 13, no. 8 (2008): 808–823.

Hill Street Blues. "Slum Enchanted Evening." Episode number 21. Directed by Michael Switzer, Jonathan Lemkin, Michael Wagner. Written by Walon Green, Robert Ward. NBC, March 27, 1986.

Hinyard, Leslie J., and Matthew W. Kreuter. "Using narrative communication as a tool for health behavior change: a conceptual, theoretical, and empirical overview." *Health Education & Behavior* 34, no. 5 (2007): 777–792. https://doi.org/10.1177/1090198106291963.

Hoffner, Cynthia, and Martha Buchanan. "Young adults' wishful identification with television characters: The role of perceived similarity and character attributes." *Media psychology* 7, no. 4 (2005): 325–351. http://dx.doi.org/10.1207/S1532785XMEP0704_2.

House. "Hunting." Episode number 7. Directed by Gloria Muzio. Written by Liz Friedman. FOX (US), November 22, 2005.

How to Get Away with Murder. "There's My Baby." Episode number 14. Directed by Stephen Williams. Written by J. C. Lee, Erika Harrison. ABC (US), March 10, 2016.

Iconis, Rosemary. "College students and HIV/AIDS awareness." *American Journal of Health Sciences* 2, no. 1 (2011): 1.

Ingold, Charles H. "Socially Desirable Responding and Self-Reported Reactions to Sex on Television." *Southwestern Mass Communication Journal* 26, no. 1 (2010).

Jemmott, Loretta S., and John B. Jemmott. "Applying the theory of reasoned action to AIDS risk behavior: condom use among black women." *Nursing research* (1991).

Johnson, Judith Ann, and Sharon Coleman. "AIDS Funding for Federal Government Programs: FY1981–FY2006." Congressional Research Service, Library of Congress, 2000.

Johnson, Malynnda A. "More Than Pop Culture: Depictions of HIV in the Media and the Effect on Viewer's Perception of Risk." *Journal of homosexuality* 60, no. 8 (2013): 1117–1142. https://doi.org/10.1080/00918369.2013.776423.

———. "Asking Numbers to Speak: Verbal Markers and Stages of Change." *Qualitative Health Research* 26, no. 13 (2016): 1761–1773. https://doi.org/10.1177/10497323166 65349.

Kaiser Family Foundation, Survey of Americans on HIV/AIDS, Conducted March 24–April 18 2006.

———. Survey of Americans on HIV/AIDS—Summary of Findings, Conducted April 2009.

———. HIV/AIDS at 30: A Public Opinion Perspective, Conducted June 2011.

Katz, E., Blumler, J., & Gurevitch, M. Utilization of mass communication by the individual. In J. Blumler & E. Katz (Eds.), *The uses of mass communication: Current perspectives on gratifications research* (pp. 19–32). Beverly Hills, CA: Sage, 1974.

Kelly, J., and S. L. Smith. "Where the girls aren't: Gender disparity saturates G-rated films [Research brief]." www.thriveoncreative.com/clients/seejane/pdfs/where.the.girls.arent.pdf (2006).

Kelman, Herbert C. "Processes of opinion change." *Public opinion quarterly* 25, no. 1 (1961): 57–78.

Kim, Janna L., C. Lynn Sorsoli, Katherine Collins, Bonnie A. Zylbergold, Deborah Schooler, and Deborah L. Tolman. "From sex to sexuality: Exposing the heterosexual script on prime-time network television." *Journal of Sex Research* 44, no. 2 (2007): 145–157. http://dx.doi.org/10.1080/00224490701263660.

Kincaid, D. Lawrence. "Drama, emotion, and cultural convergence." *Communication Theory* 12, no. 2 (2002): 136–152.

Kinsella, James. *Covering the plague: AIDS and the American media.* Rutgers University Press, 1989.

Knowles, Eric S., and Jay A. Linn, eds. *Resistance and persuasion.* Psychology Press, 2004.

Kunkel, D., Cope, K., & Colvin, C. *Sexual messages on family hour television: Content and context.* Menlo Park, CA: Kaiser Family Foundation, 1996.

Kunkel, Dale, Keren Eyal, Keli Finnerty, Erica Biely, and Edward Donnerstein. "Sex on TV 4 2005: a Kaiser Family Foundation report." (2005).

LaBrie, Joseph W., Jason Schiffman, and Mitchell Earleywine. "Expectancies specific to condom use mediate the alcohol and sexual risk relationship." *Journal of Sex Research* 39, no. 2 (2002): 145–152.

LaBrie, Joseph W., Thomas Quinlan, Jason E. Schiffman, and Mitchell E. Earleywine. "Performance of alcohol and safer sex change rulers compared with readiness to change questionnaires." *Psychology of Addictive Behaviors* 19, no. 1 (2005): 112.

Lanier, Yzette, Ted Castellanos, Roxanne Y. Barrow, Wilbert C. Jordan, Virginia Caine, and Madeline Y. Sutton. "Brief sexual histories and routine HIV/STD testing by medical providers." *AIDS Patient Care and STDs* 28, no. 3 (2014): 113–120. doi:10.1089/apc.2013.0328.

L.A. Law. "The Venus Butterfly." Episode number 9. Directed by Donald Petrie. Written by Steven Bochco, Terry Louise Fisher. NBC, November 21, 1986.

L.A. Law. "Say Goodnight, Gracie." Episode number 22. Directed by Rick Wallace. Written by Charles H. Eglee, Channing Gibson, Alan Brennert. NBC, May 21, 1992.

Law & Order: Special Victims Unit. "Quickie." Episode number 11. Directed by David Platt. Written by Ken Storer. NBC, January 6, 2010.

Lewis, John E., Maria-Jose Miguez-Burbano, and Robert M. Malow. "HIV Risk Behavior among College Students in the United States." *College Student Journal* 43, no. 2 (2009).

Lieberson, Jonathan. "The reality of AIDS." *New York Review of Books* 32, nos. 21–22 (1986): 43–48.

Life Goes On. "Last Wish." Episode number 16. Directed by Joe Pennella. Written by Bill Smitrovich. ABC (US), March 7, 1993.

Lincoln, Y. S., & Guba, E. G. (1985). "Establishing trustworthiness." In Y. S. Lincoln & E. G. Guba, *Naturalistic Inquiry* (pp. 289–331). Newbury Park: Sage Publications.

Lindlof, Thomas R., and Bryan C. Taylor. *Qualitative communication research methods.* Sage Publications, 2017.

Madhu, K. P., M. Malan, M. Engebretsen, H. Hashmi, P. Sharma, and S. Etzenhouser. "Getting the Story and Telling it Right: HIV on TV." *United Nations Educational, Scientific, and Cultural Organization (UNESCO Series on Journalism Education)* 6 (2009).

Marshall, Catherine, and Gretchen B. Rossman. *Designing qualitative research.* Sage Publications, 2014.

Martino, Steven C., Rebecca L. Collins, David E. Kanouse, Marc Elliott, and Sandra H. Berry. "Social cognitive processes mediating the relationship between exposure to television's sexual content and adolescents' sexual behavior." *Journal of Personality and Social Psychology* 89, no. 6 (2005): 914.

McGlathery, James M. *Grimms' fairy tales: A history of criticism on a popular classic*. Camden House, 1993.
McCombs, Maxwell E., and Donald L. Shaw. "The agenda-setting function of mass media." *Public Opinion Quarterly* 36, no. 2 (1972): 176–187.
McGrane, Wendy L., Eric B. Allely, and Frank J. Toth. "The use of interactive media for HIV/AIDS prevention in the military community." *Military Medicine* (1990).
McKee, Neill, Jane Bertrand, Antje Becker-Benton, and Benton Lee Becker. *Strategic communication in the HIV/AIDS epidemic*. Sage, 2004.
Meyrowitz, Joshua. "No Sense of Places." New York: Oxford University Press, 1985.
Midnight Caller. "After It Happened." Episode number 3. Directed by Mimi Leder. Written by Stephen Zito. NBC, December 13, 1988.
Miles, Matthew B., and A. Michael Huberman. *Qualitative data analysis: An expanded sourcebook*. Sage, 1994.
Moustakas, Clark. *Phenomenological research methods*. Sage, 1994.
Moloney, Gail, and Iain Walker. "Talking about transplants: Social representations and the dialectical, dilemmatic nature of organ donation and transplantation." *British Journal of Social Psychology* 41, no. 2 (2002): 299–320.
Morgan, Michael, and James Shanahan. "The state of cultivation." *Journal of Broadcasting & Electronic Media* 54, no. 2 (2010): 337–355. http://dx.doi.org/10.1080/088381510037350 18.
Morgan, Susan E. "The power of talk: African Americans' communication with family members about organ donation and its impact on the willingness to donate organs." *Journal of Social and Personal Relationships* 21, no. 1 (2004): 112–124.
Morgan, Susan E., Tyler R. Harrison, Lisa Chewning, LaShara Davis, and Mark DiCorcia. "Entertainment (mis) education: The framing of organ donation in entertainment television." *Health Communication* 22, no. 2 (2007): 143–151. http://dx.doi.org/10.1080/10410230701454114.
Morgan, Susan E., Tyler R. Harrison, Shawn D. Long, Walid A. Afifi, Michael S. Stephenson, and Tom Reichert. "Family discussions about organ donation: how the media influences opinions about donation decisions." *Clinical Transplantation* 19, no. 5 (2005): 674–682.
Moscovici, Serge. "The history and actuality of social representations." In U. Flick (Ed.), *The psychology of the social*. Cambridge, England: Cambridge University Press. (1998).
Moyer-Gusé, Emily. "Toward a theory of entertainment persuasion: Explaining the persuasive effects of entertainment-education messages." *Communication Theory* 18, no. 3 (2008): 407–425. doi: 10.1111/j.1468–2885.2008.00328.x.
Moyer-Gusé, Emily. "Extending the examination of audience involvement with media personae: Response to Brown." *Communication Theory* 25, no. 3 (2015): 284–289. https://doi.org/10.1111/comt.12071.
Moyer-Gusé, Emily, Adrienne H. Chung, and Parul Jain. "Identification with characters and discussion of taboo topics after exposure to an entertainment narrative about sexual health." *Journal of Communication* 61, no. 3 (2011): 387–406. doi: 10.1111/j.1460–2466.2011.01551.x.
Moyer-Gusé, Emily, and Robin L. Nabi. "Comparing the effects of entertainment and educational television programming on risky sexual behavior." *Health communication* 26, no. 5 (2011): 416–426.
Moyer-Gusé, Emily, Parul Jain, and Adrienne H. Chung. "Reinforcement or reactance? Examining the effect of an explicit persuasive appeal following an entertainment-education narrative." *Journal of communication* 62, no. 6 (2012): 1010–1027. doi: 10.1111/j.1460–2466.2012.01680.x
Murphy, P. Karen. "The eye of the beholder: The interplay of social and cognitive components in change." *Educational Psychologist* 42, no. 1 (2007): 41–53. DOI: 10.1080/00461520709336917.
Murphy, Sheila T., Lauren B. Frank, Joyee S. Chatterjee, and Lourdes Baezconde-Garbanati. "Narrative versus nonnarrative: The role of identification, transportation, and emotion in reducing health disparities." *Journal of Communication* 63, no. 1 (2013): 116–137. doi: 10.1111/jcom.12007.

Murphy, Sheila T., Lauren B. Frank, Meghan B. Moran, and Paula Patnoe-Woodley. "Involved, transported, or emotional? Exploring the determinants of change in knowledge, attitudes, and behavior in entertainment-education." *Journal of Communication* 61, no. 3 (2011): 407–431. doi: 10.1111/j.1460–2466.2011.01554.x.

Murphy, Sheila T., Heather J. Hether, and Victoria J. Rideout. *How Healthy is Prime Time?: An Analysis of Health Content in Popular Prime Time Television Programs*. Henry J. Kaiser Family Foundation, 2008.

Murphy, Sheila T., Lauren B. Frank, Meghan B. Moran, and Paula Patnoe-Woodley. "Involved, transported, or emotional? Exploring the determinants of change in knowledge, attitudes, and behavior in entertainment-education." *Journal of Communication* 61, no. 3 (2011): 407–431. doi: 10.1111/j.1460–2466.2011.01554.x.

NBC Universal Media, Robert Bazell, *Early Studies on AIDS.* Television Broadcast. June 17, 1982.

Neon Rider. "Saint Walt." Episode number 2. Directed by Bruce Pittman. Written by Brad Writght. CTV, 1992.

Newcomer, Susan F. "Research on Adolescent Sexual Socialization." *Gay People, Sex, and the Media* (2014): 77.

Nip/Tuck. "Erica Noughton." Episode number 1. Directed by Ryan Murphy. Written by Ryan Murphy. FX (US), June 22, 2004.

Nusbaum, Margaret R. H., and Carol D. Hamilton. "The proactive sexual health history." *American Family Physician* 66, no. 9 (2002): 1705–1722.

NYPD Blue. "Hollie and the Blowfish." Episode number 17. Directed by Davis Guggenheim, Bill Clark, David Simon. Written by David Simon. ABC (US), March 26, 1996.

Oblinger, Diana. "Boomers gen-xers millennials." *EDUCAUSE review* 500, no. 4 (2003): 37–47.

O'Donnell, Victoria. *Television criticism*. Sage Publications, 2016.

O'Leary, Ann, and Shirley Brown. "Self-efficacy and the physiological stress response." In *Self-efficacy, adaptation, and adjustment*, pp. 227–246. Boston, MA: Springer, 1995.

O'Leary, Ann, Fern Goodhart, Loretta Sweet Jemmott, and Daria Boccher-Lattimore. "Predictors of safer sex on the college campus: A social cognitive theory analysis." *Journal of American College Health* 40, no. 6 (1992): 254–263.

O'Leary, Ann, Fern Goodhart, Loretta Sweet Jemmott, and Daria Boccher-Lattimore. "Predictors of safer sex on the college campus: A social cognitive theory analysis." *Journal of American College Health* 40, no. 6 (1992): 254–263.

Opt, Susan K., and Donald A. Loffredo. "College students and HIV/AIDS: More insights on knowledge, testing, and sexual practices." *Journal of Psychology* 138, no. 5 (2004): 389–403.

Orr, Donald P., and Carl D. Langefeld. "Factors associated with condom use by sexually active male adolescents at risk for sexually transmitted disease." *Pediatrics* 91, no. 5 (1993): 873–879.

Palmgreen, Philip, Seth M. Noar, Rick S. Zimmerman, Timothy Edgar, S. Noar, and V. Freimuth. "Mass media campaigns as a tool for HIV prevention." *Communication Perspectives on HIV/AIDS for the 21st Century* (2008): 221–252.

Pardun, Carol J., Kelly Ladin L'Engle, and Jane D. Brown. "Linking exposure to outcomes: Early adolescents' consumption of sexual content in six media." *Mass communication & society* 8, no. 2 (2005): 75–91. DOI: 10.1207/s15327825mcs0802_1.

Picket Fences. "The Body Politic." Episode number 16. Directed by Mel Damski. Written by David E. Kelley. CBS, February 5, 1993.

Polacek, Georgia, N. L. Johnston, Jennifer A. Hicks, and Sara B. Oswalt. "20 Years Later and Still at Risk College Students' Knowledge, Attitudes, and Behaviors About HIV/AIDS." *Journal of Hispanic Higher Education* 6, no. 1 (2007): 73–88.

Poust, Tracy and Kinnally, Jon. "A Will & Grace-full Exit?" Interview by Lucile Scott. *POZ Magazine,* May 1, 2006.

Potter, W. James. *An analysis of thinking and research about qualitative methods*. Psychology Press, 1996.

Primack, Brian A., Erika L. Douglas, Michael J. Fine, and Madeline A. Dalton. "Exposure to sexual lyrics and sexual experience among urban adolescents." *American Journal of Preventive Medicine* 36, no. 4 (2009): 317–323. http://dx.doi.org/10.1016/j.amepre.2008.11.011.

Private Practice. "A Family Thing." Episode number 1. Directed by Mark Tinker. Written by Stacy McKee. ABC (US), October 1, 2008.

Private Practice. "Right Here, Right Now." Episode number 3. Directed by Rob Corn. Written by Dana Baratta. ABC (US), October 15, 2009.

Prochaska, James O., and Carlo C. DiClemente. "Toward a comprehensive model of change." In *Treating addictive behaviors*, pp. 3–27. Boston, MA: Springer, 1986.

Prochaska, James O., and Carlo C. DiClemente. "Stages of change in the modification of problem behaviors." *Progress in Behavior Modification* 28 (1992): 183.

Reese, S. D. 2003. "Framing public life: A bridging model for media research". In *Framing Public Life*, edited by Reese, S. D., Gandy, O. H. and Grant, A. E. 7–32. Mahwah, NJ: Lawrence Erlbaum Associates, Inc.

Reese, Stephen D., Oscar H. Gandy Jr., Oscar H. Gandy Jr., and August E. Grant, eds. *Framing public life: Perspectives on media and our understanding of the social world.* Routledge, 2001.

Regnerus, Mark. *Forbidden fruit: Sex & religion in the lives of American teenagers.* OUP USA, 2007.

Rideout, Victoria J. *Television as a health educator: A case study of* Grey's Anatomy. Henry J. Kaiser Family Foundation, 2008.

Roberts, D. F., U. G. Foehr, and Victoria Rideout. "Generation M: Media in the Lives of 8–18 Year-Olds, Kaiser Family Foundation." http://www.kff.org/entmedia/entmedia0309 05nr.cfm (2005).

Rogers, Everett M., Peter W. Vaughan, Ramadhan Swalehe, Nagesh Rao, Peer Svenkerud, and Suruchi Sood. "Effects of an entertainment-education radio soap opera on family planning behavior in Tanzania." *Studies in Family Planning* 30, no. 3 (1999): 193–211. doi: 10.1111/j.1728–4465.1999.00193.x.

Rotheram-Borus, Mary Jane, and Donna Futterman. "Promoting early detection of human immunodeficiency virus infection among adolescents." *Archives of Pediatrics & Adolescent Medicine* 154, no. 5 (2000): 435–439.

Salovey, Peter, and Alexander J. Rothman, eds. *Social psychology of health: Key readings.* Psychology Press, 2003.

Rubin, Alan M. "Parasocial Relationships." *The International Encyclopedia of Interpersonal Communication* (2016).

Rubin, Alan M., Elizabeth M. Perse, and Robert A. Powell. "Loneliness, parasocial interaction, and local television news viewing." *Human Communication Research* 12, no. 2 (1985): 155–180. doi: 10.1111/j.1468–2958.1985.tb00071.x.

Rubin, Alan M., and Mary M. Step. "Impact of motivation, attraction, and parasocial interaction on talk radio listening." *Journal of Broadcasting & Electronic Media* 44, no. 4 (2000): 635–654. http://dx.doi.org/10.1207/s15506878jobem4404_7.

Ruppel, Erin K. "Scanning health information sources: Applying and extending the comprehensive model of information seeking." *Journal of Health Communication* 21, no. 2 (2016): 208–216. http://dx.doi.org/10.1080/10810730.2015.1058438.

Salmon, C. "Setting a research agenda: Entertainment-education conference." *Centers for disease control and prevention, Office of Communication.* Retrieved March 9 (2001): 2005.

Salmon, C., K. Witte, and B. Lee. "The effectiveness of entertainment-education as media health campaigns: The effects of entertainment narrative and identification on HIV/AIDS preventive behavior." In *meeting of the International Communication Association, New York, NY.* Retrieved April, vol. 25, p. 2009. 2005.

Scheufele, Dietram A. "Framing as a theory of media effects." *Journal of Communication* 49, no. 1 (1999): 103–122.

Schwartz, H. "AIDS in the Media." Appendix to Science in the Streets: Report to the Twentieth Century Task Force on Communication of Scientific Risk. New York: Proprietary, 1984.

Scott, J. Blake. *Risky rhetoric: AIDS and the cultural practices of HIV testing.* SIU Press, 2003.

Scull, Tracy M., Christina V. Malik, and Janis B. Kupersmidt. "A media literacy education approach to teaching adolescents comprehensive sexual health education." *The Journal of Media Literacy Education* 6, no. 1 (2014): 1.

Sex and the City. "Running with Scissors." Episode number 11. Directed by Dennis Erdman. Written by Michael Patrick King. HBO, August 20, 2000.

Sheeran, Pascal, Charles Abraham, and Sheina Orbell. "Psychosocial correlates of heterosexual condom use: a meta-analysis" (1999): 90. http://dx.doi.org/10.1037/0033–2909.125.1.90.

Slater, Michael D., and Donna Rouner. "Entertainment—education and elaboration likelihood: Understanding the processing of narrative persuasion." *Communication Theory* 12, no. 2 (2002): 173–191. doi: 10.1111/j.1468–2885.2002.tb00265.x.

Sillars, Malcolm O., and Bruce E. Gronbeck. "Communication Criticism: Rhetoric, Social Codes." *Cultural Studies* (2001): 59–78.

Singhal, Arvind, Michael J. Cody, Everett M. Rogers, and Miguel Sabido, eds. *Entertainment-education and social change: History, research, and practice*. Routledge, 2003.

Singhal, Arvind, and Everett Rogers. "A theoretical agenda for entertainment-education." *Communication Theory* 12, no. 2 (2002): 117–135. doi:10.1111/j.1468–2885.2002.tb00262.x.

———. *Entertainment-education: A communication strategy for social change*. Routledge, 2012.

Smiley, Sam. "Rhetorical principles in didactic drama." *Quarterly Journal of Speech* 57, no. 2 (1971): 147–152. https://doi.org/10.1080/00335637109383055.

Smith, Kevin. *Mental Hygiene: Better Living Through Classroom Films 1945–1970*. Blast Books, 1999.

Sobo, Elisa J. "Self-disclosure and self-construction among HIV-positive people: The rhetorical uses of stereotypes and sex." *Anthropology & Medicine* 4, no. 1 (1997): 67–87. doi: 10.1080/13648470.1997.9964523.

Sood, Suruchi. "Audience involvement and entertainment—education." *Communication Theory* 12, no. 2 (2002): 153–172.

South Park. "Tonsil Trouble." Episode number 1. Directed by Trey Parker. Written by Trey Parker. Comedy Central (US), March 12, 2008.

Sparks, Glenn G. *Media effects research: A basic overview*. Nelson Education, 2015.

St. Elsewhere. "Family Feud." Episode number 15. Directed by Mark Tinker, John Masius, Tom Fontana. Written by Frank Dandridge. NBC, January 29, 1986.

Strasburger, Victor C. "Adolescents, sex, and the media: Ooooo, baby, baby—a Q & A." *Adolescent Medicine Clinics* 16, no. 2 (2005): 269.

Strasburger, Victor C., Barbara J. Wilson, and Amy B. Jordan. *Children, adolescents, and the media*. Sage, 2009.

Strauss, Anselm, and Juliet M. Corbin. *Basics of qualitative research: Grounded theory procedures and techniques*. Sage Publications, 1990.

Sutton, Michael, and Karen M. Wilson. "Shaking the Tree of Knowledge for Forbidden Fruit: Where." *Sexual teens, sexual media: Investigating media's influence on adolescent sexuality* (2001): 25.

Swain, Kristen Alley. "Approaching the quarter-century mark: AIDS coverage and research decline as infection spreads." *Critical Studies in Media Communication* 22, no. 3 (2005): 258–262. http://dx.doi.org/10.1080/07393180500206073.

Sypher, Beverly Davenport, Michelle McKinley, Samantha Ventsam, and Eliana Elias Valdeavellano. "Fostering reproductive health through entertainment-education in the Peruvian Amazon: The social construction of Bienvenida Salud!" *Communication Theory* 12, no. 2 (2002): 192–205.

Tatar, Maria. *Off with their heads!: Fairy tales and the culture of childhood*. Princeton University Press, 1992.

Taylor, Laramie D. "Effects of visual and verbal sexual television content and perceived realism on attitudes and beliefs." *Journal of Sex Research* 42, no. 2 (2005): 130–137. http://dx.doi.org/10.1080/00224490509552266.

Taylor, Laramie D., Cassandra Alexopoulos, and Jannath Ghaznavi. "Touchy Subjects: Sex in the Workplace on Broadcast, Cable, and Internet Television." *Sex Roles* 75, nos. 9–10 (2016): 476–489.

The Closer. "Head Over Heels." Episode number 7. Directed by Matt Earl Beesley. Written by Wendy West. TNT (US), July 24, 2006.

The Equalizer. "Christmas Presence." Episode number 11. Directed by Michael O'Herlihy. Written by Coleman Luck. CBS, December 16, 1987.

The Parkers. "She's Positive." Episode number 14. Directed by Tony Singletary. Written by Andrea Wiley. UPN, February 16, 2004.

Time Out: The Truth about HIV, AIDS, and You. Directed by Malcolm-Jamal Warner. Written by Thad Mumford. Paramount Studios. 1992.

Treichler, Paula A. *How to have theory in an epidemic: Cultural chronicles of AIDS*. Duke University Press, 1999.

Tsfati, Yariv, and Joseph N. Cappella. "Do people watch what they do not trust? Exploring the association between news media skepticism and exposure." *Communication Research* 30, no. 5 (2003): 504–529. https://doi.org/10.1177/0093650203253371.

Tufte, T. "Communication for social change: Struggles for visibility and voice, culture and diversity." In *International Communication Association Conference*. 2005.

Tulloch, John, and Deborah Lupton. "Television, AIDS and risk: A cultural studies approach to health communication." (1997).

Valkenburg, Patti M., and Jochen Peter. "The differential susceptibility to media effects model." *Journal of Communication* 63, no. 2 (2013): 221–243. doi: 10.1111/jcom.12024.

Vermund, Sten H., and Craig M. Wilson. "Barriers to HIV testing—where next?" *The Lancet* 360, no. 9341 (2002): 1186–1187.

Wallack, Lawrence, Lori Dorfman, David Jernigan, and Makani Themba-Nixon. *Media advocacy and public health: Power for prevention*. Sage, 1993.

Ward, L. Monique, Lauren Reed, Sarah L. Trinh, and Monica Foust. "Sexuality and entertainment media." *APA Handbook of Sexuality and Psychology* 2 (2014): 373–423.

Ward, L. Monique, and Kimberly Friedman. "Using TV as a guide: Associations between television viewing and adolescents' sexual attitudes and behavior." *Journal of Research on Adolescence* 16, no. 1 (2006): 133–156. doi: 10.1111/j.1532–7795.2006.00125.x.

Ward, L. Monique, and Rocio Rivadeneyra. "Contributions of entertainment television to adolescents' sexual attitudes and expectations: The role of viewing amount versus viewer involvement." *Journal of Sex Research* 36, no. 3 (1999): 237–249.

Weinstein, Neil D., Paul D. Grubb, and James S. Vautier. "Increasing automobile seat belt use: An intervention emphasizing risk susceptibility." *Journal of Applied Psychology* 71, no. 2 (1986): 285. http://dx.doi.org/10.1037/0021–9010.71.2.285.

Welch Cline, Rebecca J., and Sarah J. Johnson. "Mosquitoes, Doorknobs, and Sneezing, Relationships Between Homophobia and AIDS Mythology Among College Students." *Health Communication* 4, no. 4 (1992): 273–289.

Wimberly, Yolanda, Matthew Hogben, Yvonne Fry-Johnson, Sandra Moore, and Jada Moore-Ruffin. "Sexual history taking among Metro-Atlanta physicians." In *The 2006 National STD Prevention Conference*. 2006.

Wingood, Gina M., Ralph J. DiClemente, Kathy Harrington, Suzy Davies, Edward W. Hook, and M. Kim Oh. "Exposure to X-rated movies and adolescents' sexual and contraceptive-related attitudes and behaviors." *Pediatrics* 107, no. 5 (2001): 1116–1119. doi: 10.1542/peds.107.5.1116.

Without a Trace. "Expectations." Episode number 19. Directed by Rosemary Rodriguez. Written by David Rapp. CBS, April 13, 2006.

Wolitski, Richard J., Robin J. Macgowan, Donna L. Higgins, and Cynthia M. Jorgensen. "The effects of HIV counseling and testing on risk-related practices and help-seeking behavior." *AIDS Education and Prevention* 9, no. Suppl 3 (1997): 52–67.

Wong, Eric Y., Wilbert C. Jordan, David J. Malebranche, Lori L. DeLaitsch, Rebecca Abravanel, Alisha Bermudez, and Bryan P. Baugh. "HIV testing practices among black primary care physicians in the United States." *BMC Public Health* 13, no. 1 (2013): 96.

Wright, Paul J. "Mass media effects on youth sexual behavior assessing the claim for causality." *Annals of the International Communication Association* 35, no. 1 (2011): 343–385. http://dx.doi.org/10.1080/23808985.2011.11679121.

Wulfert, Edelgard, and Choi K. Wan. "Condom use: A self-efficacy model." *Health Psychology* 12, no. 5 (1993): 346.

Quick, Brian L. "Coverage of the organ donation process on *Grey's Anatomy*: The story of Denny Duquette." *Clinical Transplantation* 23, no. 6 (2009): 788–793.

Yoo, Jina H., and Yan Tian. "Effects of entertainment (mis) education: exposure to entertainment television programs and organ donation intention." *Health Communication* 26, no. 2 (2011): 147–158.

Zillmann, Dolf, and Jennings Bryant. *Selective exposure to communication*. Routledge, 2013.

Zoller, Heather M. "Health activism: Communication theory and action for social change." *Communication Theory* 15, no. 4 (2005): 341–364.

Zheng, Micha Yin, Amit Suneja, Ann Love Chou, and Monisha Arya. "Physician barriers to successful implementation of US Preventive Services Task Force routine HIV testing recommendations." *Journal of the International Association of Providers of AIDS Care (JIAPAC)* 13, no. 3 (2014): 200–205.

Zurbriggen, Eileen L., and Elizabeth M. Morgan. "Who wants to marry a millionaire? Reality dating television programs, attitudes toward sex, and sexual behaviors." *Sex Roles* 54, nos. 1–2 (2006): 1–17. doi: 10.1007/s11199–005–8865–2.

Index

About the Author

Dr. Malynnda Johnson completed her PhD in Communication at the University of Wisconsin, Milwaukee, in 2012. She is currently an Assistant Professor of Communication at Indiana State University, teaching classes in the areas of Health Communication and Media Criticism. Dr. Johnson's work focuses on the investigation of difficult conversations surrounding sex in both the media as well as the exam room. Since 2008, her work has examined social and cultural factors associated with sexual health disparities including the ways in which we talk about sex, sexual health, STIs and HIV, and sexual assault.

Experienced in conducting and overseeing research using both qualitative and quantitative methods, as well as rhetorical criticism, her work has been published in various journals, book chapters, and will soon include a co-authored health communication textbook focusing on patient advocacy.

Since beginning HIV prevention and sexual health education within the Milwaukee community she has remained dedicated to working with diverse populations. Striving to serve as a teacher and mentor in both academic and professional arenas she continues to work with young people of all ages, races, and economic backgrounds.

Twitter Handle: @MalynndaJ
Website: https://www.linkedin.com/in/malynndajohnson/